Keto Desserts

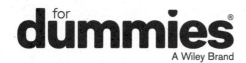

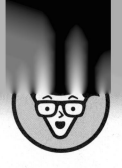

Keto Desserts

by Rami Abrams and Vicky Abrams,
authors of *Keto Diet For Dummies*

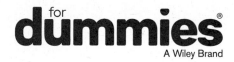

A Wiley Brand

Keto Desserts For Dummies®

Published by: **John Wiley & Sons, Inc.**, 111 River Street, Hoboken, NJ 07030-5774, www.wiley.com

Copyright © 2020 by John Wiley & Sons, Inc., Hoboken, New Jersey

Published simultaneously in Canada

For general information on our other products and services, please contact our Customer Care Department within the U.S. at 877-762-2974, outside the U.S. at 317-572-3993, or fax 317-572-4002. For technical support, please visit https://hub.wiley.com/community/support/dummies.

Wiley publishes in a variety of print and electronic formats and by print-on-demand. Some material included with standard print versions of this book may not be included in e-books or in print-on-demand. If this book refers to media such as a CD or DVD that is not included in the version you purchased, you may download this material at http://booksupport.wiley.com. For more information about Wiley products, visit www.wiley.com.

Library of Congress Control Number: 2020934300

ISBN: 978-1-119-69643-8; ISBN: 978-1-119-69648-3 (ebk); ISBN: 978-1-119-69651-3 (ebk)

Manufactured in the United States of America

V10018235_032520

Contents at a Glance

Recipes at a Glance

Table of Contents

Introduction

Welcome to the best part of low-carb dieting: desserts. The concept of keto-friendly desserts may seem counterintuitive, but that's only because you're used to thinking about sweets exclusively in terms of processed sugar. We're ready to introduce you to a whole world that includes how to lose weight, live healthier, and still be able to have desserts regularly.

In *Keto Desserts For Dummies*, we tell you about the physical, mental, and social aspects of dessert, because these cornerstones are all critical to living healthier in a sustainable way.

We firmly believe that knowledge is power, and we want to give you the freedom to go out and conquer desserts without sacrificing your health and weight loss momentum. No longer are sweets the exclusive domain of the cheat day: with this book, you can bring them into the everyday.

About This Book

One of the worst aspects of dieting is the pressure that can come from your friends, your family, social expectations, and even yourself. The best way to keep these pressures from affecting your diet goals is with knowledge and confidence, and we've found that they typically occur in that order.

Understanding how desserts fit into the ketogenic diet requires wrapping your mind around how the diet works as a biological process. Doing so helps you comprehend why certain ingredients are allowed and others are substituted. That knowledge forms the foundation of this book. Ketosis is a completely natural process your body has evolved to turn fat into energy: this works equally well with consumed fat (such as what you put in your mouth) and stored fat (for example, those few extra pounds you're tired of carrying around).

The standard American diet, or SAD — arguably the most appropriate acronym we've ever encountered — is primarily based on carbs, which the body converts into sugars. The thought that flavor comes from sugar has been ingrained in humankind's dietary thought processes for so long that many of us have lost sight of the tremendous range of delectable tastes that fat can provide. We help you rediscover how to use those building blocks to fashion an effective, sustainable diet.

The key theme we want you to focus on in this book is sustainability. Whether you decide to stay on keto long term is up to you, but you should always approach eating in such a way that you can eat well long term without having adverse side effects.

Here is an overview of the main materials we cover in this book:

>> **The adverse effects of crash dieting:** Crash dieting, even if it uses ketosis as a mechanism, only hurts your overall health. You can certainly drop a lot of weight in a short period, but we're more interested in helping you lose weight and keep it off so that you're the healthiest version of yourself. Crash dieting practices rely on rigorous eating habits and dietary restrictions that are unsustainable. When they end, the weight often comes roaring back with a vengeance; sometimes, it even brings friends! We want to help you create a diet that has space for desserts at family reunions, work functions, and other social events — simply abstaining isn't usually a long-term solution. Our previous book, *Keto For Dummies*, includes sections on appetizers, entrees, and snacks. In this book, we fully explore desserts.

>> **Substitute ingredients for baking keto desserts:** Low-carb baking involves working with ingredients that typically fall into flour alternatives, sugar replacements, and dairy substitutes. We delve deeper into them all, explain them in plain English, and advise you how and when to use them.

>> **A plethora of recipes for every kind of dessert:** The majority of this book focuses on more than 150 recipes to help you start baking your way to keto yumminess. From cakes and cookies to pies and ice cream treats, we have you covered. We also include recipes you can use for holidays.

Here are a few other guidelines to keep in mind about the recipes in this book:

>> All butter is unsalted unless otherwise stated. Margarine isn't a suitable substitute for butter.

>> All eggs are large.

>> All salt is kosher.

>> All dry ingredient measurements are level.

>> All temperatures are Fahrenheit (see the appendix to convert Fahrenheit temperatures to Celsius).

>> All lemon and lime juice is freshly squeezed.

» All Greek yogurt is full-fat yogurt.

» All dark chocolate chips are unsweetened, no sugar added. Our go-to favorite for chocolate chips is Lily's Chocolate Chips. They're perfect for keto baking because they're sweetened with erythritol and stevia.

» All protein powder is unflavored, sugar-free whey protein powder, no sugar added, low carb.

We have your back and want to help you overcome common hurdles. This handy guide sets you up for success with everything you need to know to begin making tasty keto desserts. We want you to work *with* your body, not against it!

Foolish Assumptions

We made the following assumptions about you when we were writing this book:

» You have a basic understanding of keto, but perhaps not why desserts are so crucial to sustainable success.

» You're going to face social pressures as part of your dieting journey, and these pressures often occur at events where sweets are present.

» You have a basic understanding of how to bake and cook, but you have likely not explored keto dessert recipes.

» You're open to trying new things and working with unfamiliar ingredients.

» Your overall goal is a healthier you.

No matter who you are, you can find all sorts of helpful information here.

Icons Used in This Book

If you've flipped through this book at all, you've probably noticed little pictures, called icons, in the margins. Here's what they mean:

TIP

This icon indicates good advice and information that can help keep your baking on track.

WARNING

When we discuss something that might have special dietary considerations (such as a common allergen), we make a note of it with this icon.

REMEMBER

When we make a point or offer some information that we feel you should keep with you forever, we toss in this icon.

Where to Go from Here

This book is a reference, not a tutorial. You don't have to read it from Chapter 1 to the end if you just want to get a glimpse of the hobby before you get down to the basics. Just use the table of contents or index to find the topics that interest you and go from there. Start with your needs and interests.

If you're not sure how desserts can possibly fit into keto, start with Part 1. If you have a little more background in the diet, you may want to begin with the recipes in Part 2. If you have a holiday coming up and need a themed treat, Part 3 is going to be your (low-carb) bread and butter. Perhaps the chapter on additional resources (including sites designed around dietary restrictions or keto for kids) caught your fancy. Go ahead and skip around. That's what this book is for. You can also refer to the Cheat Sheet at www.dummies.com for more helpful advice that you can review whenever you need to.

1

Understanding How Desserts Fit into Keto

Review how keto works as a natural metabolic process and how desserts fit into that picture, including how the diet works biologically to how to make the transition from a standard American diet to embracing ketosis.

Understand how dessert impacts your mental, physical, and social well-being. You don't have to skip desserts when you're on keto, and you wouldn't want to anyway.

Wrap your mind around the impact of alcohol on your diet and discover the right way and the wrong way to drink on keto. Knowing how alcohol impacts ketosis biologically helps you make the right decisions each time.

Find out how to prep your home for keto and conquer speed bumps that may get in the way by setting effective goals to give you the highest chance of success as well as common-sense strategies for preparing your kitchen if you have roommates or family members who won't be joining you.

Explore dairy, flour, and sugar alternatives and how their unique properties affect baking. We've designed these recipes to imitate the effects that you would see with wheat flour and sugar.

Replace tasty carbs with delectable fats while losing none of the flavor. In fact, as your palate recovers from a constant carb overload, you'll likely develop a deeper appreciation for more complex tastes.

Chapter **1**

Brushing Up on the Basics

Keto continues to be one of the most popular diets worldwide, and it's not showing any signs of slowing down. Although many people try it because of the fantastic weight-loss benefits it offers, just as many (if not more) people want to be on it because of how healthy the lifestyle is. That's the reason we've stayed on keto long term: we've never felt better in our lives. That's also fundamentally different from most diets, which focus on transitioning you into the body you want and then assuming you'll transition back to the way you ate before.

The keto diet is a sustainable lifestyle choice, incorporating all elements of a meal, including dessert. That concept may seem ironic because the one thing most people know about keto is that you have to avoid sugar. When you change your eating style, however, you also change how you cook. This chapter serves as your jumping-off point to see how simple enjoying delicious sweets can be while staying low-carb.

Understanding What the Keto Diet Is

The ketogenic diet is an entirely different approach toward eating than the standard American diet (SAD) currently recommends. SAD (an ironically appropriate acronym) focuses on carbohydrates as the foundation of a proper diet, with

55 percent of calories sourced from carbs, 30 percent from fat, and 15 percent from protein. When this mix is present, your body runs off of a metabolic process called *glycolysis,* where virtually all food is converted into glucose (blood sugar) for fuel. Anything you've consumed that the body doesn't immediately need is transformed into love handles, muffin tops, back rolls, and any other term used to describe stored fat.

A low-carb diet, on the other hand, is based on 65 to 75 percent of your daily calories coming from fat, 20 to 30 percent from protein, and a minuscule 5 to 10 percent from carbohydrates. When you eat like this, your body runs off a metabolic process called *ketosis,* where your body converts nearly all calories into ketone bodies, which are used for fuel. If you eat too much fat, you'll simply excrete the excess ketones through your urine.

Many people are surprised when they discover that ketosis is a completely natural metabolic process with roots in humankind's evolutionary history. The human race probably wouldn't have survived if it just had glycolysis: the ketogenic diet was what saw the human species through the hunter-gatherer stage. Although the way people eat has changed drastically since those days, the building blocks of health haven't. You'll hear many objections to keto, and we've found the best way to address these arguments is with facts, which we discuss in the following sections.

Ketosis as an evolutionary development

The basis of a ketogenic diet is a core part of human evolution. Think back a few thousand years: before refrigeration, before modern farming, before any kind of agricultural cultivation — what was life like? Humanity's hunter-gatherer ancestors subsisted off what the land provided. Common sources of carbs were fresh fruits and vegetables; they didn't have many ways to preserve these items, so they ate them whenever they were available. Gorging was a consistent way of life.

Fruits and vegetables were only available for part of the year, and it wasn't uncommon to go for significant periods without large meals. Humanity's Neolithic ancestors would gorge on carbs: the body would use what it needed at the moment and then store any additional calories as fat. That was the only real pantry they had, so it makes sense that this is how people evolved to stock it.

After a few hours, their bodies burned through the glucose they'd just consumed and began to use its glycogen stores. *Glycogen* is a more stable form of blood sugar that's stored in the muscles and liver. Depending on their activity level, they could exhaust it within a day, and the body knew it had to keep going using its stored fat. At this point, the primary metabolic pathway switched to ketosis, which is the primary way fat is converted into energy.

When they made a kill, they would gorge themselves. Massive amounts of carbs or protein would immediately switch the body back to glycolysis so that fat could be created and stored easily. When they burned through that, the body slowly transitioned back to ketosis.

Combating common objections

You may hear objections to how "natural" ketosis is — the argument generally goes that if ketosis is so natural, why does it take days to transition into it while the body can switch back to glycolysis in a single meal? That's where we need to mention a serious, potentially deadly condition known as *ketoacidosis* that occurs when high levels of glucose and high levels of ketones are both simultaneously present in the bloodstream. It can have severe negative repercussions, including death. Chapter 2 explains this condition in greater detail.

The body precludes ketoacidosis by burning through all the glucose in your system before switching to the process that generates ketones. This evolutionary master-piece is what keeps ketoacidosis from being a common experience; in fact, it's exceedingly rare. The population most at risk for this is comprised of people who have Type 1 diabetes (T1D). With this type of diabetes, the pancreas makes little or no insulin, which is required to drive glucose out of the bloodstream and into individual cells. If the body switches over to ketosis and begins generating ketones, this condition is possible.

Your digestive system naturally prefers to utilize consumed energy (for instance, food in your stomach) before resorting to stored energy, which may not seem particularly useful in the western world of today where food is readily available. Still, it was developed as an evolutionary survival mechanism that kept the fat storage tanks topped off as much as possible while telling you to continue eating regularly, even if you had excess fat.

One of the benefits of the ketogenic diet is that it keeps your body trained to consume fat for energy. When dietary fat is burned through, your digestive system automatically switches over to stored fat without a hitch. One of the most common praises we hear from keto dieters is their steady energy state throughout the day: it isn't uncommon to skip meals without experiencing any drop in energy. Your body is consistently satiated with fats and continues to burn them at a consistent rate.

THE HISTORY OF KETO

The ketogenic diet has been around for more than a century when doctors originally created it as a medical treatment. Although its original purpose was treating epileptic seizures — something it's still used for today — one of the surprising side effects was sustainable weight loss, which led to its current popularity.

Unlike many fad diets, keto has been rigorously tested by doctors and scientists, with thousands of peer-reviewed studies examining the short-, medium-, and long-term effects on both adults and children. Historically, the harshest criticism of keto has been that in a carb-obsessed society it can be difficult to adhere to.

Conversely, the benefits are numerous and well-documented. Weight loss, a decrease in insulin resistance, more consistent mental clarity, and energy throughout the day are all reasons to at least give keto a try. Quite a few low-carb advocates stay on keto long term, while many cycle on and off of it periodically. It's a flexible diet that works *with* your body, not against it. Our life wouldn't be the same without it!

Realizing the Importance of Dessert

Because carbs are out on the keto diet, you may presume that you have to avoid desserts to stay on keto. Because of this presumption, many people approach low-carb eating as if it were a crash diet: they'll make any necessary sacrifice for a brief period to lose weight, and then go back to their regular way of eating. This plan of attack will work for a short time, but it isn't the best way to approach the ketogenic diet.

REMEMBER

The benefits of the ketogenic diet extend far beyond simple weight loss. We firmly believe that keto is a lifestyle choice: it's something we've lived for years, and we couldn't be more pleased with our decision. Mental clarity, steady energy, and the ideal weight for our body types are some of the benefits we've noticed. We also aren't okay living without desserts, so one of our goals for the recipes in this book was a robust and varied sweets menu. We were able to cobble together a subpar recipe with the right macros and call it dessert, but we didn't want to have to choke it down or force our taste buds to accept something less on a regular basis. We wanted gourmet-level treats, and we didn't stop until we found them.

One of the things we hate most is seeing people go through unhealthy diet practices. *Crash dieting* is one of the most common, and is essentially an attitude; it isn't limited to a specific named diet, and we even see people approach low-carb eating in this way. This happens when someone drastically changes their eating patterns and dietary habits for a short period with a specific goal in mind (typically it's dropping a few pounds before an event), but plan to go back to their "normal" way of eating after they've achieved their goal. Crash dieting can have serious negative repercussions not only for your physical health, but also your mental and emotional well-being, especially if it involves severely undereating calories, macronutrients, and micronutrients.

Dessert is a critical component of making a sustainable lifestyle change. You're virtually cutting out an entire group of macronutrients, so you shouldn't have to cut courses out as well. Appetizers, entrees, desserts, and snacks are all part of a balanced dietary approach, and we've found that with keto. Remember that this isn't a competition to see who can torture or deprive themselves the most or a contest to see whether you can muscle your way through an unpleasant experience. Keto should always be something that directly contributes to your overall health.

Furthermore, eating isn't always about you. The majority of social events involve some kind of food, and treats are often filled with carbs you're not allowed to touch. Technically, never attending social events or choosing not to eat at them are options, but they're never choices we would want (or expect!) someone to pick. One of our motivations for creating recipes that are so good you can't tell them from the real thing is that we're very active socially and we weren't about to give that up.

Chapter 2 provides some strategies you can use when focusing on desserts and social gatherings and also shares some of our insights for relying on your support system as you continue on your keto journey.

Making the Transition to the Low-Carb Lifestyle

Mastering a new style of cooking can take a bit of effort, and it isn't a great idea to do so while you're weaning yourself off carbs at the same time. We recommend beginning to experiment with recipes a few weeks before your official diet start date. Find what works for you, create a list of favorite recipes, and you'll be good to go starting on day one.

This pre-diet experimentation period can also be the best time to introduce family and friends to keto. You're still eating the same way they are, and introducing a keto-approved dessert that everyone can enjoy is an excellent way to kick off the conversation.

Because of the tremendous difference between SAD and a low-carb approach, the first transition can be a bit difficult. Slowly increasing your fat intake while decreasing your carbs can make easing into keto much easier. Trying out new recipes to build your top ten list is a great start. Eliminating sugary treats and carb-laden snacks should be your next step: if you do this while you can still eat carbs for your main dishes, it won't be as much of a shock to your system when you make the actual switch.

Having a plan extends beyond a list of recipes, however. We go into more depth on creating a plan in Chapter 2, but here are some quick tips to get you started:

» **Write down your reasons and goals.** Doing so can help provide the motivation you need to make such a significant change.

» **Identify obstacles you'll likely face.** They can include people, events, or anything else.

» **Identify your support structure.** Take the time to write down a list of the people you can call for advice, feedback, or even encouragement when cravings get tough.

» **Think about what specific things you need to do and when.** Wrapping your mind around your situation permits you to make the right choices at the right time, which is critical to your success.

We also cover how to evaluate the contents of your current pantry, cabinets, refrigerator, and freezer, and then select replacement ingredients that work for you. If your entire household isn't making the switch, you need to keep a few special considerations in mind that can help keep stress levels low and success rates high.

You'll encounter a few "exceptions" on keto: situations where you step outside of the bounds of the diet, such as cheat meals or consuming alcohol. Knowing how to approach these scenarios allows you to enjoy their benefits and get back on track with keto as quickly as possible.

Appreciating the effects of eating dessert

If your body reacts differently to eating carbs and eating fat, it isn't any surprise that this variation extends to the world of desserts. How your digestive system treats these two macros isn't incredibly complex. Still, taking into account factors like cheat meals, whether your body is fat-adapted or not, and how intermittent fasting fits into the picture does complicate the keto diet a bit more.

As always, the more information you have, the better the decisions you can make with it. For example, cheat meals aren't necessarily bad, and they can even be necessary in certain situations. They do have specific effects on your diet though, and knowing what you're dealing with can help minimize any dietary distractions or pauses you can experience. Chapter 2 works through these issues in more detail.

Integrating alcohol into your diet

We want to help you make sustainable lifestyle choices. If you drink on occasion, you don't have to give that up; keto can still work with alcohol. However, like so many other things, it all depends on how you do it. Knowing which beers, liquors, wines, and mixers work and which ones you should avoid at all costs is crucial knowledge, especially if you're going to be in a social setting where you won't be mixing your own drinks.

Another significant consideration is how alcohol impacts your diet. The body treats alcohol like a fourth macronutrient (the first three being fat, protein, and carbohydrates), and the way your body prioritizes metabolism is fundamentally different with and without alcohol, which can have a significant negative impact on your weight-loss inertia if you don't handle drinking correctly. We dig into all of this in Chapter 2.

Discovering a New Way of Cooking

Adopting a well-rounded approach to ketogenic dieting does take some work, and it's a bit more difficult in some areas than others. For centuries, baking revolved around wheat flour and, with a few notable exceptions, yeast that required sugar to transform batter into a light, delicious product. People on the keto diet have to do without those ingredients, so certain adjustments are necessary. The good news is that alternate ingredients and substitute approaches have never been more widely available than they are today. With a little bit of work, you can transform your kitchen into a low-carb bakery that consistently produces some of the best dishes you've ever eaten.

A successful keto journey begins with understanding what you are and aren't allowed to eat. Contrary to what some may say, not all carbs are off-limits. Entire classes of carbs are both allowed and encouraged: knowing what these are and how they fit into your daily macros will make all the difference between a pleasant or unpleasant experience.

NET CARBS AND THE KETO DIET

Throughout the recipes in this book, you may see the term *net carbohydrates* or *net carbs* being used, especially in the nutritional analyses. Net carbs are what you get when you subtract any dietary fiber and sugar alcohols from the total carb count. Dietary fiber and sugar alcohols can be subtracted because they pass through the body mostly intact, having little to no effect on blood glucose. In fact, the body passes many sugar alcohols untouched, excreting them entirely. For this reason, many people can and do safely ignore the addition of sugar alcohols in their sugar-free desserts.

Note that not all sugar alcohols are created equal! Our go-to sweetener in many recipes is a sugar alcohol named erythritol. It can be found in lots of prepackaged keto desserts and is generally tolerated by most people. It has no effect on blood glucose, which is helpful to diabetics or anyone watching their sugars.

Conversely, maltitol is a sugar alcohol that actually spikes blood glucose in most people. We recommend avoiding it in baking and when purchasing snacks at your grocery store. Always read the ingredients and do your research before buying a new product.

Changing your entire approach to eating comes with a few special considerations that we briefly cover in the next several sections. As you introduce new foods into your diet, pay special attention to any that may be an allergen or intolerance. Don't get discouraged if you find foods you can't eat; there are plenty of alternatives, particularly when it comes to flour, dairy, and cooking oils.

Starting with restrictions

Your diet options will change considerably after you're on keto, and knowing whether you're dealing with food allergies or intolerances is a critical place to start. Check with your doctor and potentially an allergist/immunologist if you have any concerns at all.

Some of the more common potential allergens you'll encounter on keto are as follows:

>> Almonds

>> Cashews

>> Coconut

>> Dairy

>> Soy

TIP

If you haven't had any experience with these potential allergens, try a couple of recipes that feature them as main ingredients. Do this one at a time, not only because you want to isolate what can cause any potential symptoms, but also because as creative as we are in the kitchen, matching all those ingredients in a single dish would be a culinary masterpiece, indeed.

WARNING

If you have any reactions, stop eating the dish immediately and speak with your doctor. If you don't have a reaction, then use those ingredients if you like the way they taste. If you don't enjoy their flavor, you can find a substitute, many of which we cover in Chapter 3.

Exploring flour alternatives

Making a variety of desserts usually means you're going to be baking. If you're baking, you'll need to use flour. Traditional wheat flour is loaded with carbs, so that's out, but we're happy to report that you can use numerous alternatives that are available. The challenge lies in recreating the texture and consistency you want to have in your dessert, which can vary, so you likely won't find one replacement flour that does it all, simply because different ingredients have different properties.

Chapter 3 discusses seven replacement options, outlining their behavior, texture, consistency, and their use in conjunction with each other to create the effect you want. Some flour substitutes won't work like you want if they're used alone, but we recommend combination strategies that work well when combined with others.

Achieving the same effects as wheat flour with substitute ingredients is as much of an art as it is a science, so be prepared for some experimentation and some trial and error. Don't be discouraged if you don't get it right the first time. That's pretty common even when you're trying a new recipe without changing cooking styles entirely. If you keep trying and experimenting, we're confident that you're going to love the results.

Milking dairy replacements

The majority of dairy products are very pro-keto. Butter, sour cream, and heavy cream can be everyday staples in your kitchen. Milk, on the other hand, contains a substantial amount of lactose, which is a dairy-based sugar. You can still drink it in small quantities, but the days of pouring a full glass and chugging it with a handful of warm chocolate chip cookies are probably in the rearview mirror.

You can find quite a few milk replacement options on grocery store shelves, however. Here are some of the more popular offerings:

- » Almond milk
- » Cashew milk
- » Coconut milk
- » Flax milk
- » Heavy cream
- » Hemp milk
- » Soymilk

You can swap most of them for milk as a drinking option, but they all have slightly different effects on cooking and baking. Chapter 3 covers the characteristics of each of these options, including their taste, texture, and effects on cooking and baking. Similar to flour replacements, you'll likely end up using more than one of these substitutes, but knowing which one to use when is crucial to creating the proper baking results.

Flavoring food with fat versus carbs

The majority of people grew up with a carbohydrate-heavy diet, where every recipe was based on the presumption that fully half of the calories would come from this macro group. Keto is different in that it relies on fats rather than carbs. Fat is the foundation of flavor in keto, offering a wide variety of tastes, textures, consistencies, and effects on various dishes. We feel pretty confident saying the fat-based desserts we include in this book are every bit as tasty, if not even better, than sugar-based ones.

You can flavor your foods, desserts included, with the following ingredients, listed in alphabetical order:

- » Avocados
- » Cheese
- » Dark chocolate
- » Eggs
- » Nuts

These are just a few of the full-fat options that can cause your taste buds to virtually explode with excitement. Don't think about venturing into low-carb cooking as a journey away from carbs; instead, focus on the door that just opened to an entire world of new possibilities that's literally dripping with flavor. Refer to Chapter 3 for more tidbits about these foods.

Cooking with grease

Whether it's frying, sautéing, or simply adding it as a central ingredient in a baking recipe, cooking oils play a foundational role in supporting the keto diet. As you're figuring out how to embrace a full-fat approach to healthy eating, you can begin to eliminate some of the misconceptions about fat you've learned in American society.

Cooking with fats involves understanding several characteristics, including *smoke point* (similar to when water turns to steam, oil turns to smoke at a high enough temperature), aftertaste, and storage considerations. When cooking with fats, you should stay away from many of the oils and fats that tend to be common in SAD. Instead focus on the following list of approved oils; we delve into them more in Chapter 3:

- » Avocado oil
- » Butter
- » Extra virgin olive oil
- » Lard
- » Light olive oil
- » Sunflower seed oil

These keto-friendly alternatives give you a lot of options, and more than likely you'll end up using several different ones, depending on the effects you're trying to achieve. Don't be overwhelmed by the number of choices, though; you'll wind up with two or three main staples that you'll like and use again and again, but deciding which those are depends on the type of dishes you like, the tastes you prefer, and the way you prepare them.

Enjoying All Types of Keto Desserts

Just because you're eating keto doesn't mean you have to sacrifice your favorite kinds of dessert. From classic desserts you can serve throughout the year to celebrating special occasions, we include a wide array of keto–approved, healthy, and yummy desserts:

» **Cakes:** Don't listen to the naysayers: you can have your cake and eat it too, even on keto. In Chapter 4 we show you how to make pound cake, cheesecake, and numerous others.

» **Candies:** Candy has a well-deserved reputation for being almost completely made of sugar. We've developed multiple recipes in Chapter 5 that allow you to revel in these decadent sweets while staying on keto.

» **Pies:** Chapter 6 covers a cornerstone of baking: the art of baking pies. You're sure to find a recipe that will satisfy anyone's taste buds in this section.

» **Cookies:** From the classic chocolate chip cookie to a few new recipes you may never have tried, Chapter 7 is filled with suggestions for enjoying various kinds of cookies.

» **Ice cream/frozen treats:** Few things are more satisfying on a hot summer day than a refreshingly sweet bowl of ice cream. Chapter 8 keeps this tradition alive while helping you stay on track with keto.

» **Mug cakes and dump cakes:** While Chapter 4 covers full-sized cakes, Chapter 9 is all about individual-sized portions that are quick and easy to make.

» **Milkshakes and smoothies:** The unique texture of milkshakes and smoothies is made even more delectable on keto with a range of healthy fats that fill each sip with flavorful creaminess. Check out Chapter 10 for a milkshake or smoothie for any occasion.

» **Hot drinks:** Cold winter days are made much brighter by a steaming hot mug of your favorite beverage. Chapter 11 has several variations of coffee and cocoa in addition to a few new drinks you may never have tried.

» **Cocktails:** There's no reason why you can't enjoy the occasional alcoholic beverage on keto, and Chapter 12 gives you a great start on drinking socially while keeping it low-carb.

A NOTE ABOUT RECIPES WITH CHOCOLATE

Chocolate can definitely be part of a balanced keto diet and is used frequently in our recipes. However, you need to be sure that you're choosing the right kind of chocolate, ensuring extra carbs don't sneak into your baking.

The first rule of choosing keto chocolate is that the chocolate has no added sugars and is just pure chocolate. Carefully check the label on a bar of chocolate because only cocoa beans and cocoa butter are listed as the ingredients. If there is milk, sugar, or any other kind of syrups added to the chocolate, it likely isn't keto-friendly.

Dark chocolate is your best option, especially when it comes to baking. Choose a dark chocolate that has at least 75 percent cocoa solids (it may even go all the way up to 90 percent), which not only is perfect for a keto diet, but it's also said to be healthier, containing more flavanols that have been shown to promote heart health.

Some great chocolate brands are available on the market that we love using in keto baking. Lily's brands of chocolates are one of the best and most widely available. You can find dark chocolate chips as well as dark chocolate bars made by Lily's, and they will work perfectly in all the recipes in this book that utilize chocolate. Lily's chocolate is actually sweetened using a small amount of erythritol and stevia, both of which prevent the chocolate from being overly bitter while sticking to the keto requirements.

You can try many other brands as well, such as Lindt supreme dark (which has a very high cocoa percentage), Hershey's sugar-free, and Choc Zero, which uses a monk fruit sweetener. Just be sure to read the labels and choose a dark chocolate with no added sugars or milks. You'll be enjoying tasty chocolate treats in no time!

Embracing Natural and Artificial Sweeteners

Here we want to acquaint you with alternatives to processed sugar. The three main ones are as follows:

» **Plant-based sweeteners:** These are found in nature and either don't impact your blood glucose levels at all or do so at a very decreased level.

» **Chemical derivatives:** These sweeteners consist of various chemical compositions that affect your taste buds like sugar does, but the rest of your body reacts differently.

>> **Sugar alcohols:** These by-products of sugar fermentation occur naturally in trace amounts in various fruits and vegetables. They retain the taste of sugar but aren't metabolized in the same way, making them low-carb.

All the sweeteners we recommend are safe to eat in normal amounts. (Refer to the earlier sidebar, "Net carbs and the keto diet" to help you understand how to read the recipes' nutritional analyses in terms of sugar alcohols.) Chapter 19 discusses in detail the top ten keto-approved sweeteners.

Our personal favorites

The top three sweeteners we recommend are erythritol, monk fruit extract, and stevia. After years of experimenting with every possible ingredient and combination, we've settled on these three as our favorites.

We always recommend experimenting with a variety of ingredients to find what suits you best, but starting with these three will minimize the impact of switching from processed sugar to keto alternatives. If you don't find a perfect match immediately, don't get discouraged; try the next one on the list and move on until you find what you're looking for.

Erythritol

This sweetener is the best of the sugar alcohols. It's the closest substitute to actual sugar in terms of taste, texture, consistency, and the effects it has on baking. Erythritol doesn't affect blood sugar, making it ideal for keto and those who deal with diabetes. You can find this sweetener in either granular or powdered form, and it's sold alone or in combination with other sweeteners. Another plus: it minimizes the possibility of potential gastrointestinal side effects that other sweeteners cause and mitigates their effects even when they do show up.

Monk fruit

This is one of our absolute favorite natural products. Unlike the vast majority of fruits, these small green globes aren't sweetened by fructose, but rather by mogrosides. *Mogrosides* are antioxidants and anti-inflammatory; they promote higher energy levels and work as natural antihistamines, among numerous other benefits. Who would have thought that your sweetener would have health advantages that beat your multivitamin?

It doesn't raise your blood sugar levels at all but does have a bit of a distinct flavor. We've found that most people like it, but the aftertaste is something you'll want to consider when using it. Monk fruit extract comes in liquid form, powdered form, and powdered form combined with other sweeteners (such as an erythritol/monk fruit extract blend). Which one you use depends on what you're doing with it. We typically advise sticking with liquids if you're sweetening drinks and a monk fruit extract/erythritol blend for everything else. Pure dehydrated monk fruit extract can be challenging to mix with other ingredients, but when it's combined with erythritol, it combines in recipes effortlessly.

Stevia

This one rounds out our top three. It's derived from the leaves of the stevia plant. One of the unique properties of stevia is its ability to increase insulin production and glucose tolerance. Although you'll be limiting your glucose intake on keto, stevia is an excellent transitional sweetener if you've been diagnosed with pre-diabetes or deal with insulin resistance due to its ability to help the body stabilize in this area.

Because stevia works differently than sugar, it activates both the sweet and bitter receptors on the tongue. Depending on how sensitive their taste buds are, some people detect a bitter aftertaste. It's stable for baking and cooking, but because it's so sweet, far less of it is required, which causes the recipe to lose some of the bulk that sugar previously provided. You'll likely have to make a few additional adjustments to get the exact result you want, but cooking with stevia is definitely an option.

Dealing with pre-fab keto products

Today's busy world sometimes prevents cooking every meal from scratch, and you're often faced with tough decisions about how to maintain your diet while operating under a tough work and family schedule. Even though avoiding processed foods is generally our default advice, the decision becomes a bit tougher when dealing with dishes, ingredients, and meal replacements designed from the ground up with keto dieters in mind. Chapter 3 discusses the role of processed keto food products, including exogenous ketones and meal-replacement shakes.

Discovering Other Resources

Having a support system and additional resources at your disposal is vital to your success. We know we don't have all the answers. You can refer to other resources to expand your keto desserts knowledge to the broadest possible base.

In Chapter 20, we cover ten sites you should bookmark and visit as you continue your low-carb journey. Many of these have specific focuses, so if you're a parent, an athlete, or are dealing with a blended household (in this context, we mean a home where some people are eating low-carb and others aren't), we have a resource for you. Several of these sites cover dietary restrictions in depth: whether you're vegan, vegetarian, or have gluten, dairy, or nut allergies, you'll find a resource to cover that focus in this chapter.

Chapter **2**

Recognizing Why Desserts Are Important to Keto

The concept of *keto desserts* sounds like it's an oxymoron, ranking up there with "giant shrimp" and "deafening silence." After all, doesn't the whole concept of keto revolve around eliminating all sweets? This is where understanding the basics of how keto works (see Chapter 1) is crucial to know what desserts you can and can't eat, and more importantly, why. This chapter discusses why desserts are important psychologically, what the dietary aspects of the sweet, final dinner course are, and how you can manage or avoid common social pressures.

Making Sustainable Diet Choices

One of the biggest downfalls we see in keto dieting is approaching this eating style from the wrong perspective. So many people are looking for a quick fix in a few weeks. Perhaps they need to drop ten pounds before a wedding, reunion, or bathing suit weather, and they want to take a bit of weight off for a few months. They don't really care how it happens as long as the job gets done.

Often people end up *crash dieting,* which is broadly defined as any eating practice you use to lose weight that isn't sustainable. Keto is a sustainable lifestyle choice, and adopting this mindset is something we encourage everyone who tries the diet to do. It doesn't mean you're committing to eating this way for life; it simply means that if you wanted to, you could. If you eat a keto diet, you'll always be seeking balance. Eating sustainably keeps you out of trouble later when the cravings come, and the pounds want to creep back on.

Crash dieting — keto or not — doesn't work long term: you'll see that weight come right back on within a few weeks of reverting to your former ways of eating. More importantly, though, your body is experiencing a type of digestive torture that often resembles a light form of starvation. This puts additional stress on your organs and digestive system that can potentially lead to serious health consequences.

Even more important, though, is what it can do to you mentally. Eating disorders are a real and serious problem. They almost always begin with body image issues, and they universally include an unhealthy, unsustainable approach to eating. That's not what keto should ever be, and we're strong proponents of never adopting an eating style that you can't continue long term. Whether you choose to make keto a lifestyle or not is up to you, but you should approach it in such a way that you can keep going long term with no adverse health effects.

Dieting practices, good or bad, start with your mindset. This attitude guides your actions and determines your results. These three factors are always present: intentionally shaping them to fit your goals is often the difference between achieving them and failing to.

Comparing crash dieting and sustainable eating

Crash dieting and sustainable eating exist on opposite ends of the spectrum and are different in three main ways.

- » Your mindset
- » Your actions
- » Your results

You may find it interesting that food isn't on that list. When you change your eating habits for a short-term fix, you can go with any number of approaches that span a broad range of ingredients, food groups, and macros. Crash diets tend to resort to drastically cutting calories rather than emphasizing the quality of what you're eating, and because of how the body works, that eventually hampers your ability to lose weight at all.

The following sections explain these three differences in greater detail.

The way you look at it: Your mindset

Sustainable eating starts with the proper mindset. You're choosing to emphasize your health through what you eat, and doing so takes precedence over appearance. You'll lose weight at a slower rate, but the weight loss will be steady, and the chances of experiencing that dreaded rebound weight get significantly lower. *Rebound weight* occurs when people achieve their weight-loss goals and then revert to old patterns of eating — the same patterns that put the weight on in the first place. When you do so, it isn't surprising to see the fat you worked so hard to lose come rushing back, and sometimes it brings a few extra pounds with it.

Emphasizing health over appearance is where diet and health success begin. We've seen a popular social trend toward accepting all body types, regardless of condition. The underlying concept is fantastic: you don't have to fit anyone else's expectations of what your body should look like. Everyone is built differently, with unique strengths, weaknesses, and challenges. Everyone wants something about their bodies to be different, and most people have struggled at various times with wondering whether they're attractive enough to be accepted. We absolutely endorse not only accepting your own body but also falling in love with it.

Unfortunately, this movement has a nasty flip side. Although everyone should accept others for who they are, that doesn't mean a particular person's current state is automatically healthy. The United States is dealing with an epidemic of obesity, with nearly 40 percent of adults dealing with this condition. If we expand that demographic slightly to include people who are overweight, more than two-thirds of Americans aren't living the best life for their bodies. Accepting your body is a wonderful thing, but treating that body poorly isn't.

Choosing health over appearance is interesting because you're not really making a choice. You're just setting your priorities. Placing health first usually allows you to achieve the appearance you want, whereas making how you look your highest priority will eventually ruin both. Sustainable eating allows you to start living your best life now, without having to force yourself through 60 or 90 days of unpleasantness, only to see those results quickly disappear.

The way you respond: Your actions

The mind guides the body, and your attitude toward dieting will drive your actions. Snacking, for example, isn't bad, but like everything else you put in your body, there's a right way and a wrong way to go about it. Discover how to snack well, and you can snack for the rest of your life. Try to hold your breath and avoid all treats between meals, and you'll end up grumpy, hangry, and swan-diving into a pile of potato chips at the first opportunity.

Desserts are the same way. They're a normal part of life and a natural way of eating. Sweets are a cornerstone of social life. Cutting out this entire course is certainly possible, but doing so is usually far from easy and often involves making yourself and others uncomfortable. A much better approach is to find a sustainable way of preparing and eating desserts that allows you to achieve and maintain your ideal body shape without making you feel like a social outcast.

Turning down "bad" (carb-laden) desserts is much easier if you actually have an alternative option. For example, choosing between lava cake and keto lava cake is a far, far better choice than choosing between lava cake and nothing. Again, your dieting practices (and success) come back to what is sustainable. Take for instance the five most common New Year's resolutions, which are as follows:

>> Exercise to get in shape

>> Diet to lose weight

>> Save money

>> Eat healthier in general

>> Something for self-care

It's no coincidence that New Year's ends the official holiday season, and everyone tries to work off the pounds they gained by eating too many sweets at parties. A recent study found that nearly 11 percent of gym memberships start in January, substantially more than any other month of the year. Unfortunately, the same trends occur here as they do everywhere else in the "dietsphere" (the world of people trying to lose weight): drastic actions don't last. Social scientists have found that commitments to weight loss and health-related resolutions begin to drop off substantially a mere three weeks into January, and by the middle of February, the majority of individuals who made goals to lose weight have reverted to their old habits.

What the end goal is: The results

Depending on your personal goals, keto can address or at least facilitate four of the five of the bullets in the previous section. However, you'll only find the success you're looking for if you avoid the crash dieting mindset and subsequent actions. Results are the end goal, and you should correctly frame the outcomes you're looking for. Focus less on what you'll look like 30 days from now and more on how you'll feel, how much your health will improve, and the satisfaction you'll get by achieving the lifestyle you want through healthy eating habits.

We're obviously huge fans of the keto lifestyle, but we also know that it isn't a perfect fit for everyone, and some other approaches can be better for certain individuals, particularly when health issues are involved. One thing we're absolutely certain of, though, is that the standard American diet (SAD) is far from the best way of eating. Many people have been using this approach since childhood, and reprogramming your life can be difficult to adjust to a healthier way of eating. Approaching your results with a crash dieting mindset will only work against your long-term health.

Desserts are, surprisingly, a pretty big part of making sustainable lifestyle changes. Everyone needs treats from time to time, and many dieters use cheat meals or cheat days as a reprieve from their new lifestyle. These can be helpful techniques while you're transitioning from a SAD to keto in the first 30 or 60 days, but beyond that, cheating typically hurts your weight-loss goals more than you may think. (Chapter 1 explains how the keto diet works.)

Enjoying the journey is absolutely critical to making a sustainable shift in your health, and desserts play a critical psychological role. Because keto changes your entire approach to food preparation, it isn't like some diets where you continue eating the same things but drop your calories by 50 percent.

Dividing fat bombs and keto desserts

If you've been around keto for any length of time, you've almost certainly heard of fat bombs, the delectable treats that are filled with low-carb ingredients, focusing less on protein and carbs and heavily emphasizing fats. They can taste phenomenal and be both a delicious and nutritious snack. Needless to say, we're big fans.

A TALE OF TWO KETO DIETERS

Picture two different people: one who approaches keto as a sustainable lifestyle change and one who uses it as a short-term fix to lose weight. Both have an initial target of staying on keto for 90 days. The first person embraces keto wholeheartedly, making appetizers, entrees, soups, and desserts. If she craves something, she finds a low-carb replacement. The second person, however, doesn't see the point of slow, steady weight loss. He wants results now and is willing to adopt a far stricter approach to maximize his short-term gains: no appetizers, no desserts, nothing but the bare minimum he needs to get by. However, this plan is pretty tough, so he allows himself a single cheat meal every week.

Both dieters become fat-adapted after about five days. Their bodies have transitioned to ketosis, their stores of glucose and glycogen are depleted, and they begin burning through fat. By the end of the first week, the sustainable eater celebrates by making a keto dessert, treating herself to a low-carb fudgy chocolate truffle or strawberry short-cake. Her macros remain steady, her body stays in ketosis, and her weight loss continues uninterrupted.

However, the second dieter celebrates by having a carb-loaded cheat meal. It's only a single meal in seven days, so he doesn't believe it will affect him too much. By the end of the meal, though, his body has reverted to glycolysis and is focused on burning through the sugar he just consumed. His body stores anything beyond his immediate needs (which is quite a bit) as glycogen, replenishing the stores he spent five days depleting during his initial transition. The body's ability to store glycogen isn't unlimited, however, so the body converts some of this single cheat meal to fat, actually increasing what he's worked so hard to deplete. Because glucose binds with approximately two to three times its weight in water, he also retains more water weight. By the end of a single cheat meal, he can wipe out his weight loss from the previous week.

The two dieters begin the second week. The sustainable eater has continued an uninter-rupted course: she hasn't gained any weight back, and she loses more weight this week. The crash dieter returns to his strict regimen and spends the next two to three days convincing his body that he's actually back on keto. After he becomes fat-adapted again, he begins to lose weight. The problem is that he's now approximately ten days into keto and may very well be the same weight as when he started, but at the ten-day mark for the first dieter, she's lost four pounds.

Over time, the second dieter's system will become better at switching back to ketosis more quickly, but losing a day, or even two, of progress for every carb-laden cheat meal is extremely common. The first dieter continues chugging along, losing weight less dras-tically than the crash dieter, but the progress is steady and uninterrupted. At the end of the 90 days, sustainable dieters will have transitioned, discovering a variety of recipes that taste just as good — or better — than their SAD counterparts. The first dieter lost 30 pounds and is happy continuing on to day 91 and beyond. The crash dieter lost 15 pounds, which isn't shabby at all, but he's been counting down the days until he can abandon this restricted way of eating and get back to normal. On day 91, he dives back into old ways of eating with a vengeance, and more than likely will gain back most of the weight he lost within the first month. By day 120, however, the sustainable eater is just as satisfied with her eating habits as he is, and she has lost another 10 pounds. Final score: the sustainable dieter lost 40 pounds, whereas the crash dieter focused on holding his breath through an unpleasant weight-loss journey lost 5.

The difference between low-carb desserts and fat bombs lies mostly in how you use them. Most people intrinsically know that they can't eat dessert all the time, but keto's emphasis on drastically increasing fat consumption can sometimes create confusion. Low-carb eating is substantially different from SAD, and many people struggle with getting enough fat, especially at first. Fat bombs can be an excellent way to increase this essential macro, but you have to be careful. These treats are often sweet, and although they're still keto-approved in moderation, even small amounts can add up, pushing your carbs over the allowable limit.

Remember that fat bombs are a snack and not the main course. They're absolutely fine in moderation, but you can't use them as meal replacements without your macros getting out of whack. Snacks are fine, as are desserts; you just need to make sure that you're eating them in moderation and staying within your macros, which is the foundation of healthy eating.

Making Desserts Social Again

If nutrition was all that mattered, everyone would probably be constrained to eating tasteless nutrition cubes. Thankfully, food is every bit as much of a social event as it is an action that's necessary for your survival. There are very few social occasions where hors d'oeuvres or desserts would be inappropriate, and when you're on keto in a carbohydrate-obsessed gathering, you'll face some difficult choices.

Don't let that get you down, though. Even difficult choices have a right option, and we want to make staying on course as easy and enjoyable as possible for you. A crucial aspect of staying on track is knowing how to use food, and particularly desserts, in a social context, which we discuss in the following sections.

Using sweets at social events to keep your diet on track

Eating desserts to stay on track with your diet may seem ironic, but that's precisely the way you should think about social gatherings and keto. Going low-carb doesn't have the same restrictions as many other diets, which rely on either an extremely limited list of permissible foods or a substantial caloric drop. Keto allows you to enjoy every course in a meal; you just have to redirect where you're getting your calories. However, rest assured that you can effectively navigate any social gathering, regardless of how many sweets are there, if you make the right decisions.

Here are some strategies you can follow:

>> **Don't attend any events.** Although this option may be appropriate in some situations as well as a convenient excuse to not attend that reunion with the side of your family tree you just can't stand, in the long term it isn't a great option. No one wants to be a shut-in for the sake of her diet, and it's something we believe is completely unnecessary.

>> **Attend, but don't eat.** Going to a social event but not eating anything at all isn't really much of an option. This choice relies on extreme levels of self-control to make it through an unpleasant situation. Few people have this level of discipline, and it isn't sustainable. Not eating can also make people feel uncomfortable when they're loading up on holiday cuisine and you're avoiding all the food.

>> **Bring a keto dessert or two.** This strategy is much better, giving you the option of eating and socializing with everyone else without having to deny yourself or create an awkward situation. After you begin making some of the recipes in this book, you'll be shocked at how delicious they are. We've found that when someone discusses "healthy desserts" or "diet desserts," what most people think of is a regular dessert without the sugar.

Trust us, we're as grossed out at the thought of sugarless flour cookies or brownies infused with spinach as you are. As professional foodies, we're not willing to accept a lower level of enjoyment just because we're choosing healthy eating. Every dessert recipe we use can stand on its own, without anyone thinking it's diet food unless you tell them.

One of the misconceptions society has is that flavor and sweetness can only come from sugar and carbs, which couldn't be further from the truth. Before the last hundred years, fat was the basis of virtually all intense flavors, only falling out of favor due to a combination of incredibly cheap sugar and erroneous nutrition information. It took us a while to figure out how to make low-carb desserts that tasted every bit as good as the original, but we've found that many of these recipes produce dishes that we enjoy more than their carb-laden counterparts.

The revelation that our "diet food" was tastier than many traditional desserts led us to one of our favorite things to do at social gatherings. We typically bring a keto dish, which is often a dessert, but we don't tell anyone that it's made differently. We simply put our eggnog cheesecake balls or chocolate peanut butter fudge on the table and let people dig in. When people find out that the dish is actually low-carb, it isn't uncommon to get a completely flabbergasted look in return — and several people have decided to try keto right then and there.

Introducing family and friends to keto

So many fad diets have been introduced over the last 50 years that people tend to automatically assume anything that's new and popular has no scientific or factual basis. We run into misconceptions about keto all the time, and occasionally it can turn into outright judgment. What someone chooses to eat shouldn't be anyone's business but his own, but it's one of the areas that unfortunately can create a lot of drama. Results are the best way to show someone that keto is different, but they'll only really listen when they see you enjoying your new lifestyle.

Anyone can torture himself and lose weight, but someone wiping drool off his face with a pained expression when seeing cake really doesn't engender much envy. Being happy with your sustainable nutrition choices while eating delicious desserts right alongside someone typically gets people asking questions, though.

This brings us to another side of social eating: avoiding negative influences. Support systems are so important when making a lifestyle change this substantial, and when family and friends view your choices negatively, it can put a damper on your enthusiasm that has nothing to do with food. We've interacted with thousands of new keto dieters who deal with this, and with rare exception, the people who view low-carb eating negatively have never had a real experience with it.

The best way to be a keto evangelist isn't by using words. You'll be able to convince some people that this is a good idea by using intelligent talking points, but the vast majority will remain skeptical. If you use their own taste buds, however . . . well, let's just say that piques interest like nothing else.

You likely don't care what Susie from Accounting feels about your diet at the office holiday party, but you're probably a bit more inclined to care about what your parents, brothers, sisters, and close friends think when you get together for a holiday gathering. These people are in your life day in and day out, and getting them on board is much more crucial. We like to use the term *keto ambassadors* anytime we're introducing people to low-carb living because that's precisely what we are.

SUCCESS IS A MINDSET

Failing at a diet virtually always involves discouragement. Remember that every single person has setbacks, unforeseen circumstances, plateaus, and any number of factors that keep them from being successful.

We've found that it's best to keep what we call a "forward-focused" mentality rather than a "backward-focused" one. If something negative happens, reflect on it long enough to know how to overcome it, and then move on. Do your best to forget about it. You can't change what happened, but you can change what you'll do next. Mistakes happen, but what you do with it is most important.

We have a friend who has tried keto repeatedly. She'll do fine for a while, but then she gets frustrated and quits after a couple of weeks. She'll try it again a few months later, only to experience similar results. Eventually, she realized that the same thing happened every time before she quit. She'd experience two "failures" in a row — they may have been accidental slip-ups, times when she forgot to plan ahead, or a moment of weakness with a piece of cake at a birthday party. None of these were huge deals, but if she ever had two of them back-to-back, she'd get so discouraged with herself that she'd abandon the diet.

When she discovered what was happening, we sat down and had a conversation about it. The worst consequences of even two slip-ups in a row was a temporary setback in her diet, perhaps lasting as long as a couple of days, but that was it. Her diet wasn't wrecked or ruined, she hadn't failed at anything, and the situation wasn't hopeless. Life had just happened. She decided to try keto again and push through it this time. If she hit two mistakes in a row, she'd call us and talk through the discouragement.

She's been on keto for nearly two years now and is completely satisfied with where low-carb dieting has brought her. Sometimes it takes the smallest things to distract you from your goals; understanding and overcoming those things can be the start of something amazing.

REMEMBER

Keto isn't a perfect fit for everyone; some individuals have health conditions or life circumstances that prevent them from eating this way. However, we genuinely believe that the ketogenic diet is what our bodies were designed for, and we love introducing this way of thinking and eating to those we care about. We've found that many of the negative beliefs people have about keto revolve around three main assumptions:

>> Low-carb food is gross.

>> You can't have anything that's sweet on keto.

>> The keto diet would be so unpleasant, so it should be called torture.

Interestingly enough, the news has reported so many success stories about keto weight loss — including a number of high-profile celebrities — that we rarely encounter someone who thinks keto won't work. Most of the objections we encounter center on how awful this restrictive way of eating must be, and they assume it's so bad that they could just never do it.

That's why we bring keto desserts to parties. When your family and close friends taste properly made low-carb desserts for the first time, more than likely they won't forget the experience anytime soon. Nothing takes the wind out of judgmental sails more quickly than people eating a second helping and then finding out that it's keto-approved. They may not immediately decide to try the diet themselves, but they'll almost certainly be more open and accepting of the fact that this is a choice you've made. That acceptance can make all the difference in your relationships and eliminate one of the biggest hurdles people encounter when trying to transition to keto.

Overcoming Diet Obstacles

Everyone faces obstacles when transitioning to a new way of eating. Even though many of these speed bumps are common, many of the challenges you face will be unique to you. What may be a showstopper for someone else can be no problem for you, and the opposite is also true. Expecting that the journey won't be easy at first is critical to ensuring that you achieve your goals.

Before you transition to keto, sit down and think through several things:

>> Why you're pursuing this

>> What your goals are

>> What obstacles you may face

>> What your support structure looks like

The main reason to think through these things isn't to focus on the negatives and get discouraged. We want you to understand the challenges so you can develop a plan to overcome them, and it's best to work through these issues before you get into any carb cravings or social pressures to change course.

Arguably the single greatest habit successful dieters have is being intentional, which begins with thinking through why you're dieting in the first place, what you want to achieve, how you're going to overcome potential roadblocks, and who is going to help you along your journey.

Outlining your reasons

Understanding your motivation to start keto shapes all your subsequent actions. The cornerstone of keto is *macros* (there are three macronutrients, or macros: fat, protein, and carbohydrates), and you should adjust them based on what you're trying to get out of it. If your goal is weight loss, your nutritional goals will be different from someone who is trying to build muscle. If you're pursuing low-carb living because of a condition like Type 2 diabetes or other health issues, your dietary makeup isn't going to be the same as someone who is cycling on and off keto for strength and conditioning.

There's no wrong answer here, and your reasons can be intensely personal. You don't need to share this information with others if you don't want to. The reason we want you to outline your reasons is so that you can be absolutely certain about why you're changing your eating and lifestyle patterns. At the end of the day, you're only accountable to yourself, and you need to know your own why.

Identifying your goals

Your motivation is what's behind you, what's propelling you forward, what will keep you going in the hardest moments. Goals, on the other hand, are the things you're striving toward: what you want to achieve, the results you want to create, and the differences you want to happen in your life. The best way to structure goals is to make them SMART. The following list explains what each letter stands for and how it relates to you:

» **Specific:** Specific goals are a necessity. Saying you want to lose weight can be achieved by an afternoon in a sauna and dropping a pound of water weight. However, knowing exactly what you're aiming for often makes the difference between discouragement, thinking that you'll never get where you want, and maintaining slow, steady progress.

» **Measurable:** To be specific, your goals need to be measurable. You don't have to limit yourself to the standard "I want to lose X number of pounds." Be creative. Define your goals in inches, or choose a certain dress or pair of pants you want to fit into. Perhaps have your cholesterol and HbA1c levels checked and then track your progress every couple of months to see how much your health is improving. There's no one-size-fits-all answer, so don't try to fit yourself into a mold you've seen other people pursue. Determine what you're trying to do, and then go after that. Whatever that is, though, if you make it measurable, your chances of achieving it skyrocket.

>> **Attainable:** As you decide how to measure your progress, make sure it's attainable. Perhaps you want to lose a lot of weight, but you're feeling pressured because you think you have to perfectly understand and structure precisely what you want to achieve from the start. Nothing could be farther from the truth. In fact, it's actually better if you don't have your end state in mind.

TIP

Concentrate on a shorter-term goal — perhaps you need to lose more than 100 pounds, so make your first milestone something like 20 or 25 pounds. Massive, overarching objectives that may take a year to achieve can actually work against you by feeling like a Mount Everest. Smaller goals give you a sense of achievement that only serves to inspire and maintain your progress.

>> **Realistic:** Being realistic is critical. Although many people can lose a pound a day at certain stages of their keto journey, this isn't the norm. Making it your goal to lose 30 pounds in 30 days is probably going to discourage you more than help. Err on the conservative side: remember, you're going for slow, steady, sustainable change. It's much better to take six months to lose 30 pounds that you're going to keep off permanently than to lose the same weight in a month and gain it right back over the next six weeks. If you reach your goals more quickly than you expected, awesome! Patience is a vital part of effective dieting practices.

>> **Time-oriented:** The flip side of patience, however, is keeping yourself focused and pursuing your goals relentlessly. There's a subtle difference between patience and apathy: you need to be willing to wait to see your dreams realized but want them enough that you're willing to work day in and day out to make that happen.

TIP

Consider creating a timeline and hold yourself to it. Be aggressive enough that you'll actually have to push yourself to achieve your goals, but practice enough self-restraint to know that you're in this keto journey for the long haul, for permanent change, and that consistent progress is far, far more important than rapid change.

When you put all these things together, you have a SMART goal. Here are a few examples we've seen in the past:

>> I weigh 200 pounds today, and I want to lose 15 pounds over the next six weeks. I want to weigh 185 by June 15.

>> I want to fit into this dress by the wedding on September 2, which is four months away.

>> I want to reduce my A1C levels from 6.7 percent to 5.5 percent in the next six months. My target date is March 1.

These goals are all specific, measurable, attainable, realistic, and time-oriented. None are impractical, and they're structured in such a way that you'll push yourself to achieve them.

REMEMBER

Make your SMART goals completely your own. Don't let anyone tell you that a target is wrong for you if you believe it's something worth achieving. Write down the goals and then post them somewhere you'll see them regularly. Doing so can go a long way toward paving the way to success.

Working with dietary restrictions

Keto, to a large degree, is all about finding replacement ingredients as you discover a new way to prepare and enjoy food. You may find that you can't stomach some common replacements (for example, soy products or almond milk), or perhaps certain artificial sweeteners don't agree with your system. That's totally fine; we've written this book so you can experiment with various replacements and annotate those changes within the recipes themselves. Chapter 3 discusses the baking and cooking properties of dairy replacements and artificial sweeteners in greater detail.

Don't get discouraged if your first attempt at a recipe doesn't turn out quite like you expect. Try to figure out what went wrong, make changes (perhaps trying a substitute ingredient), and go for it again. These sections identify some of the allergens we see in keto-approved replacements.

Soy

Soy is found in a variety of low-carb ingredients, such as soymilk and soy flour. If you have a soy allergy, you're probably already aware of it, but keep an eye out for these reactions, just in case. Although these symptoms aren't common, they're important to pay attention to. If you notice any of them, stop eating what caused it and seek medical attention immediately:

>> Tingling in the mouth

>> Hives

>> Itching

>> Swelling of the lips, face, tongue, or throat

Soymilk is a common substitute for milk, especially in baking. You'll also find this ingredient in tofu, TVP (textured vegetable protein), and several low-carb protein powders. Keto is very meat-friendly, so if you can go with an animal protein source, don't be afraid to meet your macro needs there.

Because soy is so common, watch for it in any prepared or processed foods or ingredients. Vegetable oil, canned fish and meat, deli meats, and peanut butter are low-carb inclusive but have a high likelihood of containing some soy. Carefully read the nutrition label to identify these ingredients if they're present; for anything prepared in a deli, ask the grocery store for a nutrition facts label, which allows you to see precisely what is in each dish.

Almonds

Almond allergies typically fall into two classes:

>> **Severe and life-threatening (anaphylaxis):** If you have this type, you're likely well aware of it; if you have any doubts, be sure to get checked out by a medical professional before making almonds part of your diet, particularly if you're not in the habit of using them regularly.

>> **Secondary:** This lower-grade allergy is classified as *secondary* because it has less to do with the nut itself than it does with the generic protein found in almonds. This protein is also found in birch pollen, a common cause of spring hay fever. Other sources of this same allergen are hazelnuts, walnuts, some pipped fruits (referring to small, hard seeds within a fruit, such as apples, oranges, and pears), stoned fruits (such as cherries and peaches), and certain vegetables like carrots and celery. If you suffer from seasonal allergies or have reactions to any of these other foods, check with your doctor to see how severe and far-reaching the allergy is.

Keto dieters commonly encounter almonds in almond milk, almond flour, and almond extract in baking. Although alternate options for milk and flour are widely available, some people are still tempted to use almond extract because there isn't a great replacement for this flavor. If you or someone for whom you're preparing food has an almond allergy, put extract on the no-go list. Even though the amounts you're using in any given recipe are relatively small, they're extremely concentrated. The best replacement for almond extract is vanilla extract: it has similar properties and a pleasant flavor that works well with the vast majority of desserts. Its flavor isn't as strong as almond extract, so if you use vanilla as a substitute, a general rule is to double the amount the recipe calls for.

Dairy

Many forms of dairy support the keto lifestyle and are widely used. Unfortunately, dairy can negatively affect people in two main ways:

>> **Allergic to dairy:** Dairy is one of the most common allergies, with up to 3 percent of people experiencing the condition. With dairy allergies, the body believes it's fighting off foreign invaders, and symptoms include rashes, hives,

congestion, and coughing. They can even be life-threatening, with some individuals experiencing trouble breathing and loss of consciousness. If anyone who will be enjoying your cooking deals with dairy allergies, be sure to use replacement options and avoid dairy altogether. We're happy to report that it's relatively easy to find alternatives, regardless of what form of dairy a recipe calls for.

>> **Lactose intolerance:** A related condition is lactose intolerance, which is even more common: up to 20 percent of adults experience this issue, and it's more likely in individuals of Asian, African, or Native American descent. Intolerance has to do with the digestive system: someone who is lactose intolerant doesn't naturally make *lactase,* the enzyme that's required to digest lactose. Instead of being broken down in the stomach and small intestine, undigested lactose moves into the colon, where it causes bloating and gas as bacteria breaks it down. This condition isn't dangerous, but it isn't a pleasant one either by any means.

The good news is that lactose is actually the sugar in milk (which you don't want on keto) and is removed or minimized in many low-carb dairy products, such as aged hard cheeses (parmesan, Swiss, and cheddar are common examples), Greek yogurt, and butter.

Cashews

Cashew allergies fall into two main categories:

>> **Isolated:** *Isolated* allergies mean that the condition is limited to cashews themselves,

>> **Extended:** *Extended* allergies can include all tree nuts, such as walnuts and pistachios.

Symptoms commonly occur in three areas:

>> **Skin symptoms (for example, rash):** Approximately 50 percent of allergy sufferers experience these.

>> **Respiratory symptoms (throat swelling and difficulty breathing):** About 25 percent of cases experience these.

>> **Intestinal symptoms (diarrhea, gas, and bloat):** They occur between 15 and 20 percent of the time.

REMEMBER

Nearly one-third of children are allergic to pistachios. If someone in your life has this condition, be aware that the issue can extend to cashew milk and cashew flour. Some medical authorities believe that if you're allergic to any kind of nut, you should avoid all nuts just to be safe. Other allergists disagree, stating that consuming nuts that aren't included in your allergen class can improve overall quality of life. Be aware that there are differing opinions on the subject, and check with your doctor to be certain in your particular case.

Coconut

Although coconut allergies are relatively rare, coconut is a very common ingredient in low-carb baking. It's also found in everything from cosmetics and moisturizers to shampoo and soap, so if you have this kind of allergy, you're likely already aware of it. If a recipe calls for coconut flour and you decide to replace it with an alternate option, be aware that coconut is far more absorbent than most of its fellows, so you'll likely need to make adjustments with your liquid ingredients to achieve the same effect.

Dealing with carb cravings

Regardless of how committed you are to the keto diet, at some point or another, you're going to have cravings for some carbohydrate-loaded dish. Having a plan in place ready to deal with those cravings is essential. When you face those cravings, consider these three approaches:

>> Remove the temptation.

>> Practice monk-level discipline.

>> Create a low-carb alternative.

REMEMBER

Removing the temptation and staying disciplined aren't the easiest strategies. What we find works best is creating low-carb alternatives so you can still enjoy healthy versions of what you're craving. Carb cravings are far from fun, but proper preparation and planning can mitigate or even outright prevent the majority of the struggles you'll face in these areas. Cravings are going to be far more common when you transition at the beginning of your diet, so don't hesitate to indulge in low-carb desserts more commonly than you typically would during this time. It's much better to stay on track with the type of food you should be eating and stray slightly outside of your macros than it is to wreck your diet by eating food you shouldn't have in the first place.

To handle those carb cravings, we suggest you put together a plan with low-carb alternatives as part of the plan. The following is an excellent start:

1. **Make a list of all the baked goods, desserts, and carb-heavy treats you enjoy.**

   As with many things in life, preparation is half the battle. Create the list before you start keto; otherwise, you may find yourself salivating on the paper as you write a list of your favorite indulgences.

2. **Search for alternative, keto-approved recipes after you make your list and begin working proactively with them.**

   You're fine to eat dessert daily as long as it fits within your macros, and having that psychological relief can go a long way toward ensuring victory.

3. **Prepare your kitchen to go low-carb.**

   The ideal situation is for everyone in the household to go keto together, which means you can toss or give away all the carbs in your pantry. However, we often find that one or more people in a household won't be transitioning to the diet, which means all those temptations stay right there in the kitchen. Chapter 3 discusses how you can organize your kitchen in a blended household with keto and non-keto dieters.

4. **Go shopping.**

   Make a list of all the ingredients you'll need to create your low-carb replacements and stock your newly reorganized kitchen with them. You want to have these on hand to deal with cravings as soon as possible after they appear.

5. **Practice makes perfect.**

   Try your selected recipes before you actually need them so you can decide which you like and which you don't. If you wait until you're on keto and the craving appears, you run the risk of a particular dish not meeting your expectations.

Low-carb desserts are crucial to satisfying those cravings and keeping you on track. Cheat meals can substantially slow your weight-loss momentum, and eating a keto-approved dessert every day is much better than denying yourself, living an ascetic life for six days, and then loading up on sugary treats once a week.

Understanding and fighting side effects

Transitioning from a SAD to a low-carb lifestyle can be quite an adjustment, and it isn't uncommon to experience unpleasant side effects. A few of these can be serious, whereas the vast majority of side effects are simply unpleasant and typically pass quickly.

Dehydration

Glucose and glycogen bond strongly with water, which means the more carb by-products you have in your system, the more water you're retaining. Dieters who are new to keto often lose five to seven pounds in the first week as their bodies exhaust glucose supplies and take a substantial amount of water with it. This news is excellent for anyone dealing with *edema* (excess water retention) and is generally good news for everyone. During the transition, though, fluid loss can also translate to electrolyte depletion, so take notice of related symptoms.

Dehydration can cause dizziness, rapid rises in heart rate, and lethargy and lack of energy. In extreme cases, chronic dehydration can lead to a higher incidence of kidney stones. Cramps are also a common side effect; if you have these, focus on rehydration and specifically aim to replenish your magnesium and potassium levels. The best way to do so is consume whole foods because nature typically presents these vital minerals in the appropriate ratios and levels for your body to use. However, if you're already experiencing cramps, a low-carb sports drink can prove very valuable.

Keto flu

Low-carb-induced dehydration can lead to the *keto flu*, arguably the most common side effect people experience when starting this diet. Symptoms include

- ❯❯ Brain fog and difficulty concentrating
- ❯❯ Gut issues like indigestion, constipation, and even diarrhea
- ❯❯ Headaches
- ❯❯ Insomnia
- ❯❯ Intense fatigue
- ❯❯ Muscle aches and weakness

Normal body adjustment

Although dehydration is a trigger for keto flu, you may be completely hydrated and still have to work through this stage because your body is adjusting to an entirely different way of eating than you're used to. Although keto is completely natural and utilizes a healthy metabolic pathway, the digestive mechanisms that turn fat into energy may be a bit dormant after decades of not being used. The enzymes and hormones your body relies on can take a bit of time to get used to, so expect your body to be a bit disoriented for a while. The good news is that these symptoms typically resolve themselves within a few days.

The best way to prevent (and fight) dehydration is to make sure you're drinking plenty of fluid and replenishing the vitamins and minerals you're losing. Sodium, potassium, and magnesium are the most common electrolytes transitioning dieters lose, and you can usually replace them by salting your food to flavor and drinking low/no-carb sports drinks. Supplementation isn't required in most cases, but check with your doctor if you have any concerns.

Constipation

One of the primary functions of your colon is to remove water from solid waste, creating stools and resulting in regular bowel movements. When you're dehydrated, the colon continues to pull water from fecal matter, and you end up with a much harder stool. Constipation isn't a pleasant experience and staying hydrated minimizes the chances you'll experience it.

If nature does come calling and you can't answer, consider adding MCT oil to your diet. MCTs assist your body in ketosis and also help to lubricate your digestive system. A popular method is to add it to your morning coffee. This type of coffee has become very popular and is our favorite way to drink java. Although recipes vary, the core concept is adding butter or ghee to coffee and blending it to create a delicious, foamy latte.

Diarrhea

On the other side of the digestive spectrum, your bowels can occasionally get away from you. This experience is equally unpleasant and one you want to eliminate as quickly as possible. To do so, remove any food items that contribute to this condition. Common culprits include sugar alcohols, such as erythritol and xylitol. Artificial sweeteners that end in "-ol" are typically sugar alcohols, and consuming large amounts can loosen your stools considerably. Knowing which sweeteners your body accepts and which it rejects is another excellent reason to try out keto dishes before making an abrupt transition.

You may also be consuming too much MCT oil. It's an excellent nutritional resource in moderation, but you can get too much of certain fats. If diarrhea becomes a problem, reduce your MCT oil and sugar alcohol intake, which often corrects the problem within a day or two if they're the cause. At that point, you can slowly begin increasing your levels back to where you want them to be.

REMEMBER

You may not be doing anything wrong. Your body's fat-burning enzymes are likely at very low levels, and it takes a while to ramp up production. In the meantime, you aren't used to taking in so much fat; what you can't use, you pass on. In the same way that a wet sponge soaks up far more liquid than a dry sponge, your body has to ease into utilizing fat for its energy needs.

If you've had your gallbladder removed, you're at a higher risk of experiencing diarrhea. This organ is responsible for storing bile, which is packed with enzymes that break down fat rather than just pass it through the system, and it will take your system longer to adjust to your changing macronutrient inputs.

Hunger

Hunger is a common side effect. Even though low-carb dieting doesn't require extreme caloric deficits and allows you to eat as much as you need to, the hunger you'll deal with is more psychological than physical, particularly if you've made a sudden transition. You may look at a plate full of food that's both low-carb and absolutely delicious and see a meal that isn't appetizing at all. The more strongly ingrained carb-heavy eating habits are, the more difficult the transition will be.

Keto breath

A relatively common side effect is what's known as keto breath. One of the by-products of using fat as fuel is excess acetone in your body, which is expelled through the lungs. Your tongue may feel fuzzy with an almost metallic taste in your mouth, or you may experience something as pleasant as slightly fruity breath.

As your digestive system becomes more efficient at utilizing fat, this issue typically goes away on its own. In the meantime, chew on sugar-free gum, mint leaves, or cinnamon bark, which are excellent, keto-approved ways to freshen your breath.

Making the transition easier

Transitioning from glycolysis to ketosis was easy for our hunter-gatherer ancestors — they'd been doing it for their entire lives. The transition can be more difficult today, primarily because most people have been on nearly uninterrupted glycolysis for decades. Here are several strategies that can help make the transition easier.

Transitioning slowly

We typically recommend switching to keto over several days, slowly increasing the fat content of your food while decreasing your carb intake. Doing so allows you to focus on eating right but gives you a psychological out if you need it. Define your transition period beforehand and limit it to what you decided; otherwise, your mind will always find an excuse to extend it, which will delay your results and create frustration.

Planning your menu

Finding keto recipes that you like is also an excellent preparatory step. It's difficult enough to change your entire eating style without making each dish for the first time as you're in the middle of the transition. Find appetizers, entrees, snacks, and desserts that are low-carb and fit into your macros. Try them out, keep the ones you like, and make any necessary cooking or baking adjustments beforehand. You'll experience much more stability in your diet if you have a list of foods you can count on.

Treating yourself

The more pleasant you make your transition, the more likely you are to stick with keto and experience all the benefits it can bring to your life. Even though you can muscle your way through it, you don't need to. The recipes in this book are a testament to the fact that sacrificing carbs doesn't mean surrendering flavor by any means.

Preparing for work

Beyond the physical and psychological side, be on the lookout for social and lifestyle side effects. For example, if you pack your lunch for work, think through the options of types of food you can prepare beforehand and either eat cold or heat in a microwave. Having a list of recipes you love doesn't do you any good if you dislike them as leftovers, so this consideration is important for working adults.

Eating out

If you regularly eat out, review the menus of the restaurants you frequent and find options beforehand. Waiting to do this in the moment can create intense pressure. If you're trying to converse with friends and colleagues while mentally deconstructing every menu option at the same time you're smelling the delicious scent of fried potatoes as it drifts from the kitchen, you're probably not going to feel good about the outcome.

Many restaurants provide not only their menu, but also comprehensive nutrition facts on their websites. We suggest you go through a restaurant's website before you visit and keep a list of default keto options on your phone. We also suggest you be honest with yourself. For example, many dieters fixate on the "no fast food while I'm losing weight" mindset. Even though we wholeheartedly endorse this excellent idea, we also know that the chances of life circumstances forcing you into a fast food restaurant eventually are pretty high. Even if you don't foresee using it, knowing the low-carb choices you'll make — along with any exceptions you have to request beforehand — can only serve to increase the odds of your diet's success. If you never need to use it, great! If you do, then you're already prepared.

Working with friends and family

Knowing how close friends and family will react is also important. For some reason, people feel very free to criticize the nutritional choices others make, and dealing with a lot of judgment and negative social pressures isn't helpful. You can't control the reactions of others, but you can have those conversations beforehand and know how they'll react. Knowing is half the battle and allows you to decide which individuals you'll avoid at certain times and who you'll go to for support and encouragement when you have rough moments. Refer to the earlier section "Introducing family and friends to keto" for more information.

Looking ahead

Take a close look at your calendar and review it for upcoming appointments, engagements, and events where non-keto food will be present. Major holidays and traditions can be difficult to overcome in the moment but are much simpler if you have a plan in place beforehand. Check out the earlier section, "Making Desserts Social Again" for more information.

Watching for ketoacidosis

Ketoacidosis is an extremely rare but potentially fatal condition that can correlate to the keto diet. It occurs when you experience high levels of blood glucose and ketones simultaneously. Because *glycolysis* (the way your body handles a high-carb diet) and *ketosis* (the way your body handles a low-carb diet) are mutually exclusive, this condition is very rare. It most commonly occurs in individuals with Type 1 diabetes (T1D), whose bodies can't produce insulin to deal with blood glucose. If you're on keto simultaneously, your body can create a perfect storm with severe consequences.

Even less commonly, ketoacidosis can be brought on by extreme amounts of exercise, starvation conditions, severe illness, and alcohol abuse. If you're active but not obsessive, eating regularly, and staying healthy, you can mitigate your chances of experiencing a non-T1D ketoacidosis experience.

Using social pressures positively

Peer pressure can be positive as well as negative, and you can do the following to increase your support levels:

>> **Consider finding a friend or family member to share the journey with you.** A diet buddy can be an excellent source of encouragement when you have hard moments, intense cravings, or experience plateaus. Friends can also recommend favorite low-carb recipes, help you troubleshoot any health

hiccups from a peer perspective, and celebrate your milestones and achievements with you.

» **Check out social media for keto support groups.** If you don't have someone locally or if you want a broader base of support, check out social media. You can find them on Instagram, Facebook, Twitter, Reddit, and virtually every other online platform. These groups are excellent resources when you inevitably bump up against a cooking, macros, or health question and want to pick the brain of someone who is much farther along than you are. You don't have to go through this alone.

» **Discuss your expectations.** Open communication and expectation management are crucial. Occasionally you'll encounter that one antagonist who seems to make it his life's mission to degrade your fitness journey, which can be incredibly frustrating. However, you'll likely find that people often aren't as closed to the idea of your going keto as you assume they'll be. Head off any awkward moments at family dinners, reunions, and celebrations by letting people know ahead of time what your restrictions are and then tell them you're bringing a dish to share.

Keto can be an incredibly positive social experience, filled with encouragement and exploration into new areas of nutrition and ways of cooking. It can also be a source of discouragement, relationship strain, and isolation — the difference often lies in how you approach it. You have every reason in the world to bring your entire social network along for the journey (even if they aren't sharing in the meals), so embrace this positive life change and take the people you love with you.

Understanding What Happens When You Eat Dessert

Knowing what happens when carbohydrate–laden desserts enter your body and how that differs from keto desserts is eye opening. This understanding certainly helps you make more informed decisions when temptation is present. These sections explain in greater detail what your body does after you consume desserts, how it's different between glycolysis and ketosis, and how to leverage this knowledge to give you the best keto diet experience possible.

Understanding how the body reacts to a non-keto dessert

After someone eats a high–carb meal, the body responds in the following way to digest the food:

1. **Stomach acid immediately begins to break each bite down into macronutrients.**

2. **These molecules then pass to the small intestine where enzymes break down sugar into glucose, which is released into the bloodstream.**

3. **The sugary molecules travel to muscles and organs to provide energy at the cellular level; however, glucose can't enter cells on its own.**

4. **In order to actually get the energy to the cells, the pancreas releases insulin, which binds with glucose and drives it through cell walls, where it can be utilized.**

   When normal levels of glucose are present, the body exists in *homeostasis:* it produces exactly how much insulin is needed, and the body's systems run like clockwork. Unfortunately, the amount of sugar people consume on a daily basis is far more than the human body needs. Americans average 17 teaspoons of sugar per day. That doesn't sound like a lot until you run the math and realize that equals 57 pounds a year, which is basically the size of your average 7-year-old.

   When that much glucose is present, the pancreas is consistently overworked and can wear out over time. If the cells have all the glucose they need, they ignore insulin's knocking on the door, communicating that it should carry the energy to cells down the line that may need it more. If a person maintains high levels of blood sugar for extended periods of time, the cells become used to ignoring these signals, creating a condition known as *insulin resistance.* It takes more and more insulin to force glucose through cell walls, which requires a corresponding increase in insulin production, making the situation that much worse for your pancreas. These conditions often lead to Type 2 diabetes.

5. **If all a person's cells are full of glucose, the body converts as much as it can into glycogen, which can be quickly converted into glucose if the body exhausts its resources at the cellular level.**

   Glycogen is mainly stored in the muscles and liver, and a person doesn't have an unlimited capacity to absorb it; typically 120 grams, or about 4 ounces, is all a person can hold. Any glycogen beyond these levels is converted into fat.

This adds up over time. For individuals on SAD, glucose intake rarely slows down, which means the body never even has the opportunity to go into ketosis and burn fat. All its needs are met through blood sugar, it stores the remainder, and people are stuck wondering why their pants never fit.

Seeing how your body reacts to a keto dessert

When you eat a low-carb keto dessert, something entirely different happens. First, you're likely fat-adapted at this point, so the body is already relying on fat as its primary energy source. The majority of the sweetness in low-carb dishes comes from artificial sweeteners, and the effects they have on the body vary. For example, monk fruit's sweetness comes from mogrosides, not fructose, as is the case for other fruits. If you're using this, your blood sugar will hardly experience a bump, although your taste buds are just as pleased as if you had eaten carbs. Some sugar alcohols will slightly increase your blood glucose, although at a much lower rate than what you'd see on SAD. Regardless, if you're staying within your macros, there is so little blood sugar that the body utilizes it quickly and then immediately transitions back to relying on fat.

When blood glucose is perpetually low, the body turns to breaking down fat via a process known as *ketosis.* Fat molecules are split into fatty acids, which are further broken down into ketone bodies. *Ketones* are an alternative fuel source that doesn't require insulin to pass through cell walls, so the pancreas sits by and rests, watching the body take care of itself with minimal input required.

The body always uses consumed fat before stored fat, so after you take a bite of a delectable fat bomb, your stomach instantly goes to work to generate ketone bodies. They're passed to the bloodstream, reach the cells that need them, pass through the cell walls, and are used as energy. The kicker comes when you realize what happens with excess ketone bodies. Instead of being stored as fat, like the body does with glucose, excess ketones are excreted from the body via urine.

Saying you can't get fat by eating fat may be somewhat counterintuitive, but that's a pretty fair representation of what happens. The problem is introduced when the body is so perpetually saturated with carbs that it never switches from glycolysis to ketosis, and any excess calories you consume find their way to your waistline. When you're fat-adapted, excess calories generally pass through your urine and go away.

Pitting glycolysis against ketosis

You may be wondering what happens when the two approaches in the previous two sections are combined. In other words, how does eating a sugary dessert affect a fat-adapted person, and how does eating a fat-filled decadent keto treat affect someone in the middle of glycolysis?

If your body is saturated with glucose, it never gets the chance to break down the fat you consumed. Consumed fat is converted into glucose (because your body is on the glycolysis track), passed to the bloodstream, and any excess (which will probably be a lot) is reconverted into stored fat. Eating fat can make you fat, but only if you're eating so many carbs that you're blocking the fat from being burned.

On the other hand, when someone on the ketogenic diet has a cheat meal or dessert, the body detects the presence of carbs and quickly reverts from ketosis to glycolysis. Your cells use what they can, your muscles and liver store what glycogen they can, and then depending on how much you ate, excess calories are converted into fat and stored. The body can hold up to 4 ounces of glycogen, and with each molecule binding to three or four water molecules, you can easily gain a pound of weight. The good news is this isn't a pound of fat and will be relatively easy to get rid of, but it's interesting to know that a single, sizeable portion of dessert can literally add a pound of weight to your body.

You'll continue to run on glycolysis until your blood sugar and glycogen stores have been exhausted, at which point you'll transition back to ketosis. How long that takes depends on a variety of factors: it can be as short as six hours or as long as a few days. The important thing to understand is that your body isn't actively burning fat at this stage. Even if you didn't eat enough to store any new fat, you've interrupted the fat-burning machine that is now you, and it can take days to get back on track.

Comprehending the role of intermittent fasting

Intermittent fasting (IF) is a popular practice with low-carb dieters because it accentuates your weight-loss efforts nicely. Because the body always utilizes consumed fat before stored fat, if you're eating every four hours, you're constantly satisfying your needs, and the body never needs to dip into its reserves (for example, your waistline). IF restricts eating windows to a certain period of time: some people only eat during a four-hour window, whereas others prefer a six- or eight-hour time frame. Whenever you're not eating, the body is still trucking along on ketosis, but your stomach is empty. Your cells aren't getting any more energy from there, so you automatically switch to stored fat without even realizing it.

IF gives you a much larger window when your digestive system is going into your reserves to meet its needs, The interesting thing is that after you become fat-adapted, you're rarely hungry. When you're operating off glycolysis and burn through your glucose/glycogen stores, the body is just waiting on more glucose — it doesn't rapidly switch to ketosis. This is where feelings of "hangriness" come from. With ketosis, however, the body is already burning fat, so switching to stored fat and continuing at an uninterrupted energy state is absolutely normal.

REMEMBER

IF allows you to get back on track more quickly if you do decide to indulge in carbs because it forces your body to burn through the glucose without being interrupted by any freshly consumed food. If you do cheat, a small fast can be the quickest way to get back on track. If you're fat-adapted and eat a keto dessert that fits within your macros, guess what happens? Absolutely nothing. Your body is already primed to use the fat, and a dessert that's within your macro limits is no different from everything else you're eating. It's a pretty amazing system.

Reconciling Alcohol and Keto

In addition to carbs, protein, and fat, a fourth macronutrient, at least as far as your liver is concerned, is alcohol. As far as keto is concerned, every alcoholic drink contains two main substances: the actual alcohol molecules themselves and everything else. The body processes everything else according to its nutritional composition; it's no different from how the digestive system handles orange juice or other sweet drinks. These sections focus on alcohol in greater detail.

Understanding alcohol as a fourth macro

Your body views alcohol as a fourth, toxic macronutrient. It wants to get rid of the alcohol badly, so you unconsciously stop all other metabolic processes, and the liver places a priority order on metabolizing alcohol. Alcohol isn't going to add pounds to your waistline, but the effect it has on your digestive system certainly can. If your body isn't doing anything but focusing on the alcohol, it isn't breaking down food into energy and can store much of it for later use, which introduces fat into the mix.

At the very least, even if you're making smart choices with your mixers, you're not eating any of the unhealthy food that often accompanies alcohol, and you go right back to keto when you're done, you've still interrupted ketosis, and temporarily halted the forward momentum you had. Alcohol also dehydrates you, which can introduce other unpleasant issues. Alcohol isn't forbidden on keto, by any means, but consuming it does come at a cost. That's perfectly fine as long as you're aware and have budgeted for it with your macros. You just need to know what you're getting into.

If you're going to drink, do it right — with the least possible amount of impact on your weight-loss goals.

Classifying the types

Different types of alcohol have various effects on the body and your digestive processes. Some of these variations have to do with the liquid itself — beer has far more carbs than vodka, for example — whereas the rest of the changes come from *how* you drink it — mixing a drink with low-carb tonic water is much better than using soda. Here we discuss how to adjust your alcohol consumption to align it with your diet goals.

Liquor

Generally speaking, liquor is the least disruptive alcoholic option for your system. It doesn't contain as many calories as wine or beer and has a more instantaneous effect, which typically means you'll stop drinking sooner. The best options are whiskey, vodka, rum, gin, and tequila, which are all carb-free. However, liquor is typically encased in some kind of mixer, the majority of which are heavy on the carbs, and you don't want to do that.

Look for keto-approved mixers such as seltzer water, diet tonic water, or low-carb margarita mix. The previously mentioned liquors are carb-free, but flavored variants (such as mango vodka or coconut rum) have additives that can add a substantial amount of sugar. Make sure that you know the total calorie and macros count of whatever you're drinking; don't focus exclusively on either the mix or the alcohol.

Wines

Wine can be a great option, but stick with the dry wines. Red options include Cabernet, Sauvignon, Pinot Noir, and Merlot, while keto-approved white wines are Pinot Grigio, Champagne, Sauvignon Blanc, and Chardonnay. Stay away from the sweet options like Moscato, port, sangria, Zinfandel, and dessert wines. Remember that wines also contain calories, so you'll need to keep track of the calories to stay on track with your diet.

Beer

Beer typically has about 3 grams of carbs per 12-ounce serving if you're choosing a light option. Brewers have come leaps and bounds in their pursuit of preserving taste while decreasing calories, and a number of good options exist on the market today. Read the labels or look up specific beer nutrition online and decide what to drink based on what you enjoy and how much space you have left in your macro limits.

WARNING

Keep in mind that alcohol consumption often triggers cravings while simultaneously lowering your self-control. When you consider the kinds of carb-laden fried foods that are often served in bars, it can be a recipe for a keto train wreck. There's no reason it has to be that way, however, as long as you know what your options are and have a plan to stay on track.

Chapter **3**

Identifying Common Keto Dessert Cooking Techniques

You can easily understand keto from a conceptual perspective: excess carbs cause your body to store fat, while burning fat has the opposite effect. Even wrapping your mind around the metabolic basis of the diet and how it works is relatively straightforward. Where most people trip up is in the nitty-gritty, day-to-day, rubber-meets-the-road of keto. How do you prepare food this way?

Desserts are no exception, requiring a complete mindset refresh. What do you use instead of wheat flour? How do you get the same effects if you have to avoid some dairy products? Where does the sweetness come from in carb-free baking? These are excellent questions, and we answer each in turn. This chapter gives you the lowdown on basics for cooking keto desserts.

Preparing Your Kitchen for Keto

The traditional American pantry is loaded with carb-heavy ingredients. Although some are easy to spot (that five-pound bag of sugar, for example), others are a bit more nebulous. Figuring out what you need to add to your kitchen to cook keto can be overwhelming, but we have your back. These sections spell out what you can do to prep your kitchen so you're ready to prepare your keto desserts (and other keto foods).

Understanding your goal: Differentiating between net and total carbs

The cornerstone of keto is a concept called *macronutrients*, which are essentially macronutrients in food: fat, protein, and carbohydrates. The vast majority of food fits into one of these three groups of macros, as they're commonly referred to. The standard American diet (SAD) consists of 30 to 35 percent fat, 15 to 20 percent protein, and 50 to 55 percent carbs. The ketogenic diet turns this around, with 65 to 75 percent fat, 20 to 30 percent protein, and 5 to 10 percent carbs. Limiting carbs is what will push you into ketosis.

When you track your macros, remember that not all carbs are created equally. You can divide this macro into two main groups:

>> **Net carbs:** Your hard macro limit in this area is based on *net carbs,* which are the sugars that actually make it through your digestive system and impact your blood sugar levels. You want to keep these low: get too high, and your body will begin to switch from ketosis to glycolysis, which pretty much defeats the purpose of the diet.

>> **Total carbs:** *Total carbs* are a bit more complicated. They include all net carbs, of course, but you also find a fair number of nutrients that are technically carbohydrates but don't impact you in the same way. For example, take sugar alcohols, which look like carbs, taste like carbs, and are classified as carbs, but the majority of them only give your blood sugar levels a minor bump — if they affect it at all. You can find out more details in Chapter 19, where we discuss all the major artificial sweeteners you'll encounter, along with their properties.

TIP

When preparing your kitchen for keto, focus on cutting out sugars. When you see "sugars" on a nutrition label, it counts toward net carbs, but when you see "sugar alcohol," you can ignore those grams as if they didn't exist.

TIP

Find a keto calculator online to give you a precise breakdown of your macronutrient goals and limits. Knowing your daily carb budget allows you to evaluate your nutrition labels with a critical eye and make easy judgment calls on what to keep and what to eliminate. As a handy guide, 25 grams of net carbs is a common baseline.

Finding carbs you don't have to count

In addition to sugar alcohols, another source of carbs that you don't need to count are those derived from fiber. Fiber is great for digestion, metabolism, and stool regularity. Fiber also helps by making you feel fuller and not providing many calories, which helps with calorie control. The two types of fiber are

>> **Soluble:** This type of fiber dissolves in water and can have beneficial effects on metabolism and digestion. It can slow down digestion and can help you feel fuller.

Familiar sources of soluble fiber include

- Avocado

- Broccoli

- Cauliflower

- Pecans

- Raspberries

>> **Insoluble:** This type of fiber attracts water into your stool and makes it softer and easier to pass, reducing strain on your bowel. It improves stool regularity and promotes bowel health.

REMEMBER

Depending on the dish, you can potentially reduce the carbs listed on the nutrition facts label by more than half. Doing so is a game changer and can substantially expand your food options. For example, a whopping 53 percent of the carbs in raspberries are dietary fiber; these berries can revolutionize your keto dessert game.

Organizing a blended household

When everyone in your household is transitioning to keto, preparing your kitchen for low-carb cooking is simple. Sugars get the boot and fats get the priority. You perform one, sweeping reorganization and you're done.

However, not everyone in your household may be transitioning to keto. One or more people in your house may plan to continue with a standard American diet (SAD), which gives you a few additional considerations.

Create two separate shopping lists

You need to have the ingredients on hand to cook in two very different styles. One of the cornerstones of the lowfat craze of the '90s, which many people are still feeling the effects of, is the assumption that fat makes you fat. That's only true in a specific set of circumstances; when you're consuming so many carbohydrates that your body never switches to burning fat, it stores all those extra calories in your body's "pantry" (for instance, your waistline). In this case, lowfat options do decrease the amount of weight you're likely to gain. Keto is different from a lowfat diet because it allows you to embrace the full flavor and nutritional benefits of fat, so these two approaches can require separate shopping lists.

Be prepared

Bags full of potato chips aren't what the keto doctor called for, and even things as seemingly innocuous as the wrong kinds of nuts can wreak havoc on your diet plans. Habits are foundational aspects of life, and they can be tremendously powerful tools. The flip side, however, is that it's extremely easy to go on autopilot in the kitchen, which is why having a plan is so crucial. Otherwise, you'll find yourself reaching for whatever sounds good when you're hungry, and that often will be foods you shouldn't eat.

Physically organize your cabinets and fridge

Organizing both your fridge and cabinets is critical, particularly if someone in your household isn't on keto and is still indulging in carbs. The best approach we've found is to physically separate the cabinets, dedicating some to keto and some to carbs. Having two different baking cabinets may seem redundant, but you'll find that doing so will go a long way toward decreasing stress and improving your chances of dietary success if you don't have to reevaluate each ingredient every time you open a cabinet door.

In the fridge, consider alternating shelves or dedicating a shelf to carbs only. Many of the ingredients in cold storage go both ways (for example, your produce, meat, and cheese sections likely won't change much), but you'll want to isolate some items that you may instinctively grab, like high-carb condiments.

Some ingredients are easy to categorize: anything that has loads of carbs in it doesn't go in the keto cabinet or shelf. However, numerous items can go either way. In these cases, it's always better to put anything that's keto-friendly in the keto cabinet and reserve the forbidden area for the things you can't eat. The reason is simple: anyone in your household who isn't eating keto can eat everything you have, whereas you have a list of things that aren't allowed. If you follow this organization system, you'll end up with two or three forbidden areas, and everything else will be open to you. If you put the shared items in the forbidden section, however, you'll risk carb temptations every time you open that cabinet or drawer.

TIP

Dedicate a Saturday to this task because organizing everything can be a bit of a project. Work through all your food items and check each nutrition label. Not all your food will have nutrition facts, so have your phone or a computer handy to look online for information that's missing.

You'll need some rough guidelines to decide what is and isn't keto-friendly. Start by taking your max net carbs (assume it's 25 grams) and divide it by three, one for each meal of the day. This gives you roughly 8.3 grams of net carbs per meal. Any single food item that is 8 grams per serving or higher goes in the forbidden pile. If you're spending your entire carb allotment for a meal on a single ingredient, it's virtually guaranteed that you'll go over your carb limits.

Purging all processed foods

Avoiding processed foods is virtually always a better choice than indulging in them, but we're realistic. We understand that completely eliminating everything that falls into this category is rarely practical. However, you can minimize the amount of processed ingredients you use, starting with removing them from your menu and kitchen. Be prepared for an adjustment period because processed food makes your work in the kitchen much easier, and that convenience isn't fun to overcome. The flip side is that cooking with natural foods is worth it.

A significant reason to avoid processed food is something called *calorie availability*, which refers to how easily accessible food is to be used as energy. Digestion isn't a passive process, and everything from chewing to breaking food down in your stomach to passing it through your GI tract takes work, which burns calories. The nutrition facts printed on a label display what nutritionists refer to as a *net calorie count*, because it takes into account how many calories the body will burn to digest the food you're eating; the true calorie count is higher.

Processed foods offer a premium in convenience because much of the work has already been done for you. That doesn't stop on the kitchen counter, though, and this efficiency continues through the digestive process. Unfortunately, what you're saving here isn't time; it's calories. Many of the chemical bonds in processed foods have already been broken, effectively "predigesting" the food. Your body doesn't work as hard, it doesn't utilize as many calories as the label presumed, and you end up consuming more than the label suggests because processed food has higher calorie availability.

To give you an idea of what 50 calories looks like, these are all rough equivalents:

>> One baby cheese

>> Two teaspoons of peanut butter

>> Two crackers

>> Half of one banana

>> Seven almonds

>> One inch of a cold cut sandwich

>> Four potato chips

>> One buffalo chicken wing

>> Half of one tortilla

You're obviously dealing with tiny amounts, and that's how you can picture the difference between processed and natural foods. A pound of fat is equal to 3,500 calories. You'll eat 21 meals over the course of a week. Unconsciously adding even 50 calories per meal can cut your weight-loss efforts by a full third.

Another reason to get rid of processed food and eat natural food is that the type of fat you consume is different. Not all fat is created equal, and trans fat can be on the naughty list. There are two primary types of trans fat:

>> **Naturally occurring:** This kind is typically found in meat and milk products, and they aren't a problem on keto.

>> **Artificial:** Artificial trans fats are created in an industrial process where hydrogen is added to oil to make it more solid. This process is called hydrogenation. If you see "hydrogenated" or "partially-hydrogenated" on an ingredients label, you want to stay away from it.

Processed foods also contain additives, which aren't always bad, but there are a few that can negatively impact weight-loss efforts. Here are several of the top additives you should keep avoid:

Monosodium glutamate (MSG)

MSG is one of the most common additives in savory dishes. Multiple studies have demonstrated a correlation between its consumption and weight gain, which is an excellent reason to minimize the amount that you eat. Some people can also experience headaches, sweating, and numbness from consuming too much, although this experience isn't widespread.

Food coloring

Food producers commonly use artificial coloring to brighten or accentuate colors in foods, particularly processed foods that will sit on a shelf or in a freezer for long periods and lose some of their natural color. Some consumers have raised concerns about the potential correlation between long-term consumption and elevated cancer rates, but this link hasn't been proven, and the FDA considers food coloring to be safe. However, some people do experience heightened allergic reactions when regularly consuming food dyes.

Food producers use artificial coloring to cover up something to make it more palatable. Many processed foods have been cooked at high temperatures, which eliminates many of the vitamins and minerals you should be getting. Using artificial coloring to make food appear fresher can give you a false sense of security in how good and balanced your diet is. Human beings are biologically programmed to find bright, vibrant colors appealing in our food, which is an excellent incentive to use different, fresh ingredients in a variety of dishes.

When your food is colored, however, it's a bit of a false advertisement and can conceal flaws or shortcomings in your dietary approach.

Sodium nitrite

Sodium nitrite is used in processed meats to inhibit bacterial growth while preserving natural reddish-pink color. One of the benefits of low-carb dieting is an increased capacity to handle sodium, and adding liberal amounts of salt to your food isn't much of a problem. Sodium nitrite is a bit different from regular sodium, however, because when exposed to high heat, sodium nitrite can convert to *nitrosamine*, which is known as a carcinogen.

When consumed in moderate amounts, sodium nitrite isn't much of an issue. However, some keto dieters increase their intake of processed fatty meats because it fits in conveniently with their macro limits. Bacon and sausage, in particular, contain high amounts of this chemical. Be careful of eating too much processed meat because the health repercussions go beyond simple macros.

Natural and artificial sweeteners

This category of additives is pretty broad and covers virtually every sweetener that isn't straight sugar. Some are good for you (for example, monk fruit extract), whereas others have been shown to contribute to higher rates of headaches and memory loss (for example, aspartame). Chapter 19 discusses a number of sweeteners in greater detail, but the lesson to take away is that when you make your own keto desserts, you can control the type of sweeteners you use, and therefore the effects they have on your body.

Carrageenan

This additive is a thickener and preservative that is widely used in numerous food products, including almond milk, cottage cheese, and sugar-free coffee creamers — all which you're likely to encounter on the keto diet. One of the effects of elevated carrageenan consumption is higher-than-normal levels of fasting blood sugar, which can actively combat the effects you're trying to achieve with keto. It can also contribute to elevated levels of systemic inflammation, which has a host of adverse effects. You don't need to be paranoid, but it's a reason to emphasize home cooking and fresh foods over processed products.

Sodium benzoate (SB)

Sodium benzoate is found in carbonated drinks and salad dressings. If you're regularly consuming sugar-free energy drinks, for example, you may be matching your macros, but you're also consuming higher amounts of this chemical. Several studies have shown a link between SB and attention deficit hyper disorder. When combined with vitamin C, SB can also act as a carcinogen. Even if it fits within your macro limits, minimizing your consumption of carbonated beverages is a good idea.

Artificial flavoring

Artificial flavoring uses various chemicals to imitate natural flavors. Several studies have found correlations between artificial flavoring and decreased red blood cell production, inhibited cell division, and toxicity to bone marrow cells. The good news is that these studies utilized much higher levels of artificial flavoring than you'll likely ever consume, so this news shouldn't keep you up at night.

WARNING

A more likely negative repercussion is how you're conditioning your body to react to flavors. One of the most fascinating aspects of your digestive hormones is that your body can create cravings for foods high in a vitamin or mineral that's lacking in your diet, which is a phenomenal checks-and-balances system to keep you on track. Unfortunately, this system is subject to conditioning, which is when you train your body (intentionally or not) to want something else, which is why people crave carbs. Your body doesn't need those carbs, but you've so thoroughly trained yourself to want carbs that you occasionally feel like you can't control yourself. Training your body to associate an artificial taste with a food that doesn't have the same nutrients as the original flavor can throw this internal guidance system out of whack. You may begin to crave foods that aren't providing the nutrients you need, which can unbalance your system. It's always better to eat the food you're actually craving rather than an artificial version of it.

EVEN PROS NEED SOME TIME TO ADJUST

One of our friends is a baker who loves to improvise in the kitchen. She rarely needs to reference a recipe; she just seems to have a sense of precisely what is needed at any given point. The first time she tried keto, she only lasted a few days. She found that her intuition wasn't working the way she was used to.

A few months later, she was ready to give keto another try. She researched numerous flour and sweetener alternatives, knew their properties, and went into the kitchen determined to experience success. Even though this time was better, she eventually became frustrated by how often her baked goods didn't behave the way she wanted them to. We talked through various possibilities, and that's when we made a crucial discovery.

She hadn't been using recipes.

She was so used to being able to create whatever she wanted that she hadn't taken the time to familiarize herself with some established keto recipes. We encouraged her to give it a shot, and she did. Her experience was immediately different, and her baking began to work out like she expected. Not every venture was a success, but her satisfaction skyrocketed.

After several weeks, she began to go off-script. This time, however, she was able to create like she wanted. Discovering the properties of the substitutes she was using, the combinations that worked best, and ways she could tweak her baking times took a bit more time. As soon as she was used to this new way of baking, however, she was able to return to what she'd always loved. Sometimes it's like that. We've done a lot of prep work beforehand to minimize the amount of trial and error you have to do, so when in doubt, just go back to the recipe. Eventually, you'll master the low-carb approach to baked goods and never look back.

Finding Flour Substitutes

Baking requires flour, but traditional sources of grains (such as wheat or rice) are high in carbs, requiring you to find suitable substitutes. Wheat flour is an incredibly flexible ingredient and has been a cornerstone of food prep ever since the Agricultural Revolution occurred. As a result, the majority of our recipes are designed with the unique properties of wheat flour in mind, and no universal replacement can replicate all its features. However, you can typically get pretty close with various combinations of the following flour substitutes. Knowing the properties of the flour you're using can help you understand how to fit it into this new realm of baking you're about to experience.

If you live in a rural area, finding appropriate substitutes at smaller grocery stores can be difficult. The popularity of Internet-based shopping may just solve this problem for you: you can order online from a variety of major retailers.

Almond flour and almond meal

Almond flour is first boiled to remove the skins, then ground into powder, whereas almond meal is made from nuts that were ground with their skins intact, resulting in a courser texture. Each is appropriate to use, depending on the kind of results you want to see.

Both are packed with vitamins and minerals, low in carbs, and high in both healthy fats and fiber. They're also high in magnesium, which is beneficial to everyone but can be particularly helpful with people who have Type 2 diabetes. Scientists estimate that between 25 and 38 percent of those with Type 2 diabetes have a magnesium deficiency, which can increase resting blood sugar levels and insulin resistance. Correcting this mineral deficiency can accentuate keto's beneficial results for those individuals who deal with this condition. Almond meal and flour are also gluten-free, so if you have a gluten allergy, they're great to use.

Almond flour is one of the easiest substitutes to use and can often replace wheat flour without any other substitutions or complicated measurements. Almond flour is substantially heavier than wheat flour, resulting in baked goods that are flatter and denser. Although calories are less of a consideration on keto than other diets, note that almonds contain about 60 percent more calories than equivalent amounts of wheat. The good news is that even though wheat flour is comprised of relatively empty calories, almond flour is packed with nutrients that make up for the caloric increase.

Coconut flour

Coconut flour is low in carbs and high in both protein and fiber, making it an excellent fit for low-carb macro levels. It's gluten-free and packed with the good stuff: two tablespoons of coconut flour has 1.5 grams of fat, 3 grams of protein, and 5 grams of fiber. It's also rich in manganese, a nutrient that supports bone health and is used in multiple biological processes within your body.

The downside of this flour substitute is that it's incredibly absorbent and tends to have a drying effect on baked goods. If you don't compensate for this property adequately, you'll end up with dry, crumbly products that have you craving milk. Here are a couple ways to mitigate the gritty texture:

>> **Sift the flour thoroughly before mixing it.** Unlike almond flour, coconut flour shouldn't be used as a 1:1 replacement. Instead, use approximately one-quarter of the amount of flour that's recommended in a wheat-based recipe and make up the rest of the bulk with other flour substitutes. Experiment with various flour combinations, using coconut flour in conjunction with others we mention in this chapter to create the right effect.

>> **Use plenty of eggs in conjunction with coconut flour.** The protein in egg whites helps stabilize the structure, whereas the yolks provide the additional moisture that's needed. Separating the eggs first also underscores these properties, allowing you to beat the egg whites until they hold stiff peaks, emphasizing their cohesive nature. Every quarter cup of coconut flour usually requires an additional egg to create the effect you need.

We mention flax meal here because although it is meal, it's much more useful as a liquid replacement than a flour alternative. One cup of ground flaxseed can replace ⅓ cup of oil or butter. Flax meal is also an excellent resource if you're vegan because you can use it as an egg substitute. The overall result is a product that's slightly denser, chewier, gummier, and browns a bit more easily than when using eggs. Two main types of flaxseed are golden and brown. Both have similar properties and identical nutrition profiles, and you can use them interchangeably.

Flaxseed has a hard coating that's designed by nature to be as impervious as possible, so it should be ground into meal to maximize its benefits. Otherwise, you'll find that many of the seeds pass through your entire digestive system without being digested. You can use a coffee grinder to turn flax seeds into meal right before you're ready to use it.

Sunflower seed flour

Sunflower seed flour has properties comparable to almond flour, making it a possible substitute if you have nut allergies. It's rich in fiber and protein and has a pleasant, mildly sweet flavor. The major issue with this alternative is that it's relatively high in carbs, with approximately 20 grams of net carbs per cup.

TIP

You can't find this flour on many store shelves, but you can easily make it at home using a food processor or coffee grinder. Pulse until the seeds have reached a powdery consistency and then stop immediately. Because of the high oil content, blending too much can quickly transform it into sunflower seed butter rather than flour. You'll also want to use it fresh, because storing it in powder form can cause the oils to go rancid relatively quickly. As a side note, if you use this flour with baking soda, you'll see tiny green specks in your final products, which is a result of the chemical reaction between these two substances and is perfectly safe to eat.

Pumpkin seed flour

Pumpkin seed flour has been increasing in popularity among low-carb dieters due to its high fat content (approximately 50 percent of pumpkin seed is comprised of healthy fats). It's relatively low in carbs, with approximately 14 grams per 1 cup/130 gram serving. This material has similar properties to wheat flour in many regards and can be used as an approximate replacement for almond flour in many recipes, although its high oil content makes it a poor choice for a sole source of flour. Most alternative bakers recommend using pumpkin seed flour for no more than 50 percent of flour mass in a given recipe.

Psyllium husk

Psyllium husk is a vital material to reference as a binding agent. In wheat flour recipes, gluten serves to thicken dough, trapping air bubbles, and producing light and fluffy baked goods. Alternative flours tend to be denser, but adding psyllium husk can mitigate this effect significantly. Because it's a binding agent, you can use it in drier flours like coconut flour that tend to be crumbly.

Selecting the Right Milk Replacements

Dairy tends to be keto-friendly for the most part, with products like sour cream, butter, and heavy whipping cream forming a cornerstone of keto cooking. Unfortunately, the one dairy product that's least likely to be a frequent visitor to your keto cabinet is milk because of the relatively high sugar content: lactose. As a result, you need to expand your culinary options in this area. Here are some great milk replacements:

>> **Heavy whipping cream** is the first option to consider. It's low-carb, keto-approved, and an excellent source of healthy fats. It does require a bit of adjustment to use as a milk substitute, however, primarily due to the high fat content. Depending on what kind of milk you get, the fat content will vary between 1 and 4 percent, whereas heavy whipping cream typically contains 36 to 38 percent fat. Consider reducing the amount of butter or shortening the recipe calls for to compensate for this additional richness.

REMEMBER

Milk also relies on proteins that add lightness and structure to a finished baking good. If you replace it with cream, consider adding additional egg whites to create more body and combat the heaviness introduced by the added fat. If you find that your products are still too dense and oily, add the whole egg: yolks emulsify the extra fat in cream, creating an effect that more closely resembles milk in baked goods.

REMEMBER

» **Almond milk** exists on the other end of the spectrum. Although you can use it as a 1:1 replacement for milk, it has a low fat content that you can compensate with additional butter, shortening, or heavy whipping cream.

Another thing to keep in mind is that baking soda is alkaline and acts as a leavening agent by reacting with the acid in milk. Almond milk lacks this acidity, so if the recipe uses baking soda, you'll need to add a couple teaspoons of lemon juice or vinegar for every cup of milk you use to achieve the same effects.

» **Coconut milk** offers another easy-to-use alternative for milk and can be substituted in a 1:1 ratio. If you need additional thickness, consider using coconut cream instead of coconut milk (the difference between these two products lies in different coconut to water ratios). This alternative does impart a noticeable coconut flavor to the finished product. Depending on what you're making, that can be a good or a bad thing. Many desserts benefit from a hint of coconut, but it varies, so keep this property in mind. Always purchase unsweetened coconut milk; any sweeteners substantially increase the carbs in each serving.

» **Cashew milk** is a somewhat surprising alternative because cashews themselves are on the nuts-to-avoid list due to their high-carb content. When transformed into a milk replacement, however, cashew milk only contains 1 gram of net carbs per serving. This milk replacement is most frequently compared to almond milk because of its similar properties. There are a few crucial differences, however. Cashew milk has a milder, less nutty flavor, which can be beneficial in a recipe that wouldn't benefit from an almond taste. In situations where almond extract is added, however, almond milk is preferable. Cashew milk tends to be a bit sweeter than its almond counterpart, which can undoubtedly be a boon when making desserts.

» **Flax milk** is nutrient-packed and an excellent alternative to milk in many ways, but it does have significantly different cooking properties. Arguably the thinnest milk on this list, it has zero protein and is relatively lowfat, meaning you'll need to add a thickening agent to compensate. Flaxseed meal or xanthan gum can provide excellent assistance in this area, allowing the overall effect to more closely resemble how milk behaves during baking.

» **Hemp milk** has one of the highest protein contents of any milk substitute, replacing many of the properties of gluten and allowing structure and lightness you don't find with many other milk replacements. The downside is that hemp has a robust flavor that's typically better suited for savory dishes than sweet. Use it as a 1:1 replacement for milk, but remember to add an acidic element like lemon juice or vinegar if you're using baking soda.

>> **Soymilk** is one of the more popular milk substitutes on the market. If you use it, always buy the unsweetened versions, because the carb count increases drastically when sweeteners are added. You can use soymilk as a 1:1 replacement for milk, but because soymilk has approximately half of the fat of whole milk, you'll likely need to bolster the fat content with other ingredients, such as additional butter or heavy whipping cream. This absence of fat also contributes to a blander, less rich flavor profile in many baked goods, which is something to be aware of when making substitutions and other combinations.

WARNING

If you have hypothyroidism and are taking synthetic thyroid hormone, you should avoid ingesting significant amounts of soy within four hours of taking your medication. Soy is also a phytoestrogen and may cause hormone imbalances if consumed in large quantities, especially for women.

>> **Oat milk** is a popular milk alternative for many reasons but should be near the bottom of your list. It's naturally high in sugar, containing 16 grams of carbs per 1 cup/240 ml serving, making it higher carb than the milk it's replacing. It's also fat-free, meaning it's less desirable for keto and can also prove to be a bit difficult to work into many of your baking recipes. It does have a pleasant, sweet taste, so if you're relaxing your carb limits temporarily and want to emphasize these properties, you may want to consider it.

>> **Rice milk** has nearly twice the carbs of regular milk, which pretty much makes it off-limits for anyone on keto. Like oat milk, it's also very thin, requiring an additional thickening agent to replicate dairy milk's properties in baking. Rice milk should be your last resort when cooking or baking keto.

Comparing Fat and Carbs: Where the Flavor Comes From

For centuries, fat was known as the source of flavor. It was prized for its succulent decadence and the richness it contributed to sweet and savory dishes alike. That began to change when sugar became widely available during the 18th century: Great Britain alone, for example, used five times as much sugar in 1770 as it did in 1710. Over the next 300 years, sugar slowly replaced fat because of many properties that were desirable in the Industrial Age: it had a long shelf life, didn't require refrigeration, and a very consistent result could be produced in large masses.

You may notice two things missing from this list are flavor and nutrition. Fat shines in these two areas. However, fat wasn't as easy to mass produce, to preserve without refrigeration, and to store, and it began to take less and less of a priority. As far as nutrition goes, the results speak for themselves. More than 70 percent of adults in the United States are overweight or obese, with 9 percent of the adult population suffering from Type 2 diabetes. The following sections examine flavor in more detail. We let you discover the difference yourself (spoiler alert: you're going to be happy).

Looking closer at carb substitutes

You can easily get stuck in the "sugar is flavor" mindset, even if you're not consciously thinking that thought. This section covers some of the most flavorful keto-friendly ingredients that you can use in numerous dishes.

Avocados

Avocados are comprised of approximately 77 percent fat, giving them a higher fat profile than most animal products. They're excellent sources of potassium, containing 40 percent more than bananas. This green fruit is an excellent source of fiber and lowers LDL (bad) cholesterol while raising HDL (good) cholesterol. Scientists have found that people who eat avocados regularly tend to weigh less and carry less belly fat than those who don't.

Many people use bananas in smoothies to provide that rich, creamy texture that drives the stereotypical milkshake feel. You can replace bananas with avocados, and you'll find the result even creamier, with a much more decadent taste. Guacamole may be the most famous dish to center on avocados, and with the right recipe, it's peerless. You can also use avocados as replacements for sour cream (if you're avoiding dairy), as the central feature of healthy ice cream, salad dressing, and as a creamy base for different kinds of sauces.

Cheese

Cheese is packed full of nutrients, which isn't surprising, because an entire cup of milk is often required to create a thick slice of this dairy product. It's high in protein and healthy fat, low in carbs, and an important source of calcium. Vitamin B12, phosphorous, and selenium are some of the main vitamins and minerals found in cheese along with a host of other micronutrients.

Dark chocolate

You may be surprised to see dark chocolate in this list. Milk chocolate is the most common chocolate in the United States, and although it's delicious, it's also packed with sugar and void of most of the nutrients that make chocolate a keto-loving powerhouse. Even though milk chocolate only needs to contain 10 percent cacao, the floor for quality dark chocolate is a whopping 70 percent.

Approximately 65 percent of the calories in dark chocolate come from fat, making it an excellent addition to a low-carb diet. It's chock-full of fiber, and a single serving has more than half of your daily recommended allowance of manganese, iron, magnesium, and copper. This delicious concoction is so high in antioxidants that it outranks even blueberries. Studies have shown that individuals who eat dark chocolate five or more times per week cut their chances of developing cardiovascular disease by more than half.

TIP

The deep, complicated flavor of dark chocolate pairs phenomenally well with blueberries and raspberries, two of the fruits that are allowed in a low-carb diet. As you transition to a full keto diet, be sure to keep a bar or two of this fantastic ingredient in your baking cabinet at all times.

Whole eggs

Whole eggs fell out of favor during the lowfat craze of the 1990s. We're happy to see that they're making a comeback because eggs genuinely are one of nature's most incredible food contributions. If you think about it, the purpose of the egg is to provide 100 percent of the nutrients required for a developing fetus. Packed with protein, healthy fats, and a shocking number of vitamins and minerals, an egg is one of the most well-rounded food items on the planet. It's so versatile that our primary concern with eggs is that you may wear out your taste buds.

REMEMBER

Separating eggs into the white and the yolk can revolutionize your options in the kitchen. The white is almost pure protein and can be whipped into a firm, stiff texture that imparts a whole new consistency to dishes that were somewhat boring before. The yolk is packed with fat, flavor, and nutrients and is helpful in moisturizing baked dishes that employ drier flour substitutes.

Nuts

Nuts are one of the most common sources of healthy, plant-based fats and fiber, and they're also high in protein. These crunchy treats are loaded with vitamin E and magnesium along with a host of trace vitamins and minerals.

Many Americans have a relatively limited exposure to nuts. We've found that many of our friends are surprised when we introduce them to the broad range of available flavors, from sharp to smooth and soft to succulent. You can use nuts to form flour, milk, and butter, providing a wide range of options for the keto kitchen.

If you're not intimately familiar with their tastes, buy a small amount of almonds, walnuts, and macadamia nuts to start. Try them each separately to develop an appreciation for their taste and texture. Pecans, macadamia nuts, and Brazil nuts have five or fewer grams of net carbs per 100-gram serving. On the other hand, pistachios and cashews will quickly max out your total daily carb allotment with just a handful or two.

Extra virgin olive oil (EVOO)

EVOO is a must for the low-carb dieter. Another powerful source of antioxidants, it's been shown to lower blood pressure, improve cholesterol, and fight systemic inflammation. This oil is an important source of vitamins E and K as well as being loaded with healthy fats.

EVOO's high smoke point allows it to be used at high temperatures without breaking down, which is critical in the kitchen. It has a strong, savory profile, so you should default to saving it for entrees, appetizers, and dressings rather than dessert. A lighter version of olive oil, however, has a more neutral taste, allowing it to be used in delicate baking projects.

Coconut oil

Coconut oil is king when it comes to a delicate flavor that's loaded with healthy saturated fats. In fact, coconuts are the richest sources of saturated fat on earth with 90 percent of their fatty acids classified in this group. Scientists have noted that populations that consume significant amounts of coconut rarely experience cardiovascular disease. Most of the fats are medium-chain triglycerides that go straight to the liver and are converted into ketone bodies, providing a substantial boost to your dieting efforts. Because this oil has a high melting point, it's solid at room temperature and should be avoided in salad dressings and as a finishing oil.

Full-fat yogurt

Full-fat yogurt is a phenomenal addition to your keto kitchen. It's packed with healthy probiotic bacteria, and regular consumption can lead to substantial benefits in digestive health. Studies have even shown benefits in warding off cardiovascular disease and obesity. You can use it in baking or as a snack.

WARNING

Flavored yogurt is notorious for having quite a bit of added sugar, so be sure to check the labels and purchase only yogurts that are low-carb approved. This extra sugar can not only wreak havoc on your diet, but it can also negate many of the health benefits that this powerful food can have.

Fruits

Although most fruits are off-limits on a keto diet due to their high sugar levels, some fruits, especially berries, are still okay and recommended in limited quantities, including:

>> Blueberries

>> Raspberries

>> Strawberries

>> Blackberries

>> Apples (though not more than half an apple at a time)

>> Lemons

>> Limes

How carbs and fat affect the body

You can get a tremendous amount of flavor from both fat and carbohydrates, but the effects they have on your body couldn't be more different. High amounts of carbs lead to a host of health issues, including obesity, diabetes, cardiovascular disease, lower brain function, mental fog, and cancer. A diet based on glucose results in multiple mood and energy swings throughout the day, resulting in the "hangriness" many people experience after a few hours without a carb fix.

Healthy fats, on the other hand, tend to decrease your chances of obesity and heart disease drastically. Populations that consistently consume high-fat foods have statistically significant lower diabetes rates and find that cancer growth is slowed, if not often precluded. Keto dieters report steady, stable energy states throughout the day as the body seamlessly switches between consumed fat and stored fat.

The primary downside of a high-fat diet can be summarized in a single word: inconvenience. Sugar, preservatives, and other additives combine to create shelf-stable food, and in a world as busy as today, this benefit can be tremendous. Unfortunately, the trade-off for this convenience is often your health, which is why we're absolutely in love with keto. You can get all the flavor carbs provide while avoiding a substantial number of negative side effects.

Adding healthy fat into your diet

Switching to a fat-based diet requires being intentional about all your food choices until it becomes second nature, and it starts with the food that you buy. When in doubt at the grocery store, always choose the option with the higher fat content. You'll find a stark contrast in the dairy aisle in particular, where lowfat options are abundant. Avoid the skim milk and lowfat yogurt: you're not only boosting your macro levels by choosing the heavier options, but you're also adding in a tremendous amount of crucial vitamins and minerals you would otherwise be missing.

The following are many of the cooking oil options (we discuss EVOO and coconut oil earlier in this chapter). These oil options vary in flavor, smoke point, after-taste, melting point, and nutritional makeup, all which are important to understand if you're going to select the best option for a particular recipe.

>> **Light olive oil** starts at the same place EEVO does: olives are crushed into a paste and then excess water is removed, leaving the oil behind. The lighter type is treated with chemical solvents that neutralize the olive flavor, lightening both the taste and the color. A side benefit of this process is that the smoke point is increased from 325 degrees Fahrenheit in EEVO to 465 degrees with the light version, making it ideal for frying and any other high-temperature cooking processes.

>> **Avocado oil** has one of the highest smoke points of any oil at 520 degrees Fahrenheit, and if you're cooking food at temperatures higher than this, you're probably burning instead of cooking it. It's high in monounsaturated fat and has many of the health benefits whole avocados do. Use this for searing, roasting, sautéing, and as a finishing oil.

>> **Butter** is an excellent option for low-temperature sautéing, but you should avoid it for any high-temperature applications because it has a low smoke point of 300 degrees F. The flavor that butter imparts is matchless, however, so use this freely whenever you can.

>> **Lard** is a semi-soft white fat that is derived from pig fat. Although this may sound inherently unhealthy, that's only true if you believe fat is bad for you. Lard contains a substantial amount of both monounsaturated fats (MUFAs) and polyunsaturated fats (PUFAs), making it an excellent low-carb resource. It can have an even lower smoke point than butter, though, so avoid it in recipes that call for high heat.

Even though saturated fats are typically very healthy, most oils high in polyunsaturated fats and trans fats aren't. The following is a brief list of the oils you should avoid, particularly in low-carb cooking:

>> Canola oil

>> Corn oil

>> Grapeseed oil

>> Margarine

>> Peanut oil

>> Rapeseed Oil

>> Safflower oil

>> Soybean oil

>> Sunflower oil

>> Vegetable shortening

CONSIDER CHIA SEEDS

Going from a high-carb diet to a high-fat diet can be a bit of an adjustment, and newcomers to keto often struggle with knowing just what they can eat. Another great food deserves mention due to the unique texture it can impart to various desserts. Chia seeds have exploded in popularity in recent years, which is due in equal parts to their incredible health benefits and their unique texture. These tiny seeds are loaded with omega-3s, antioxidants, fiber, protein, and essential minerals. When soaked, their gelatinous texture expands your culinary options significantly, allowing you to create keto-friendly pudding easily.

You have quite a few healthy fats and oils to choose from to replace this forbidden list, with a broad range of tastes and cooking properties. You may have to try a few that you've never experienced before, but rest assured that a keto-approved oil will meet every cooking and baking need you have.

Classifying keto sweeteners

Understanding the main categories of keto sweeteners is important before you start baking. We introduce the three main types in the following sections. Each of these has different properties, carb loads, and taste profiles. Chapter 19 discusses the top ten keto sweeteners in greater detail.

Chemical sweeteners

The most popular sweeteners in the chemical category are aspartame and saccharin. Although the term *chemical* instantly conjures up a mental image of mad scientists mixing potions in a lab that will eventually ruin your health, this isn't necessarily the case. Even pure water is technically a chemical, with a proper name of dihydrogen monoxide. Although considered safe by the FDA, individuals with certain genetic disorders, sulfa allergies, and sensitivity to migraines should typically avoid this category.

Sugar alcohols

Sugar alcohols are naturally occurring compounds that are created when glucose or fructose is fermented. *Fermentation* uses sugar as a fuel to complete the process, meaning that much of the actual glucose is burned in the process, leaving a compound comparable to sugar in sweetness but from anywhere between half to zero carbohydrates depending on the sugar alcohol.

These alcohols are absorbed at a far lower rate than sugars are, meaning their impact on your blood sugar is minimized. Although that's good, it comes with a trade-off: the undigested alcohols are passed into your small intestine, where they can cause bloating and indigestion when consumed in high amounts. Scientific discovery, though, has significantly improved the use of sugar alcohols, and some of the better ones today avoid virtually all side effects in moderate amounts of consumption. Common sugar alcohols are erythritol, mannitol, sorbitol, xylitol, lactitol, and maltitol (generally anything that ends in "-ol" belongs in this category).

Plant-based sweeteners

Plant-based sweeteners include stevia and monk fruit. The taste in these products comes from sources other than fructose, and their unique properties impart a sugary flavor without raising blood sugar levels. Because they're plant-based, they do contain unique aftertastes that some people find unpleasant. The majority of individuals either can't detect them or don't find them disturbing.

Avoiding non-sugar sweeteners

Food corporations do an excellent job of framing various sweeteners as "organic," "all-natural," and "wholesome," and these adjectives aren't necessarily untrue. At the same time, processed sugar is grown from sugar cane or sugar beets, so it's completely plant-based as well, which isn't what concerns us. The primary differentiator for anyone on the keto diet is how a sweetener will impact your blood sugar. If a particular sweetener raises your blood sugar, it pushes you toward glycolysis; if it doesn't, it helps you stay in ketosis.

WARNING

Honey, agave, molasses, and maple syrup are all natural sweeteners that are recognized by the body as sugar. Consuming even minor amounts of these can drive your body out of ketosis, drastically reducing — or even eliminating — the weight loss you're pursuing. Avoid them, even if they are natural sugar substitutes.

Fitting Pre-Fab Keto Products and Supplements into the Picture

Pre-made keto products aren't necessarily inherently good or bad, but they do have costs and benefits you should weigh before deciding where they fit into your diet. One of the most popular, and controversial, low-carb products are exogenous ketones, which are ketone bodies that are produced outside of the body and then consumed in a processed form to rapidly induce ketosis. Research is still in the very early stages for this class of products, so if you decide to use them, make sure you're staying current with nutritional developments and scientific studies. All exogenous ketones are supplements that the FDA doesn't regulate.

Even though exogenous ketones can rapidly induce ketosis, they're not meant to keep you there. You can use them to kick-start the process, but the ketones you rely on should always be produced by your body from consuming a well-balanced, healthy diet. Consider *ketoacidosis*, which is a potentially deadly condition that occurs when your bloodstream has high levels of glucose and ketone bodies simultaneously. The body has built-in mechanisms to exhaust glucose and glycogen stores before transitioning to ketosis, which prevents even the possibility of ketoacidosis the vast majority of the time. Flooding your bloodstream with ketones without first exhausting your blood glucose has the potential for creating harmful conditions, so talk with your doctor if you're considering using these.

Keto-focused meal-replacement shakes are becoming more and more popular. We've looked at the macros for a number of them, and if they fit into your diet parameters, go for it! Remember, however, that meal-replacement shakes are a convenient quick fix and aren't designed to replace real food you prepare at home. Just because they're keto doesn't mean they don't have many of the downsides of processed foods that we cover earlier in this chapter.

REMEMBER

One of the major mistakes we see a lot of beginning dieters make is to begin to look for supplements automatically. Ideally, you'll be able to get every bit of the nutrition you need, from macronutrients to trace minerals, from a well-balanced diet. However, that isn't always the case, and this can be partially due to anything from unique allergies and medical conditions to absolutely hating the taste of a certain type of food. In these cases, supplementation can be not only helpful, but necessary.

REMEMBER

The primary thing we tell people about supplements is that they're supplements. You should only look into them when you notice that your diet is creating a deficit in certain nutritional areas, and you should only use a supplement as long as it's absolutely necessary. Supplementing as an assumption can create significant imbalances in your system that, at the least, prove disruptive to your weight-loss goals, and at worst, can create medical hardships you would have avoided otherwise.

If you eat a well-balanced, low-carb diet, supplementation is typically only needed on a temporary basis when you encounter life circumstances (such as pregnancy or seasonal allergies) that require a short-term adjustment.

2

Healthy and Guilt-Free Keto Desserts and Drinks

Celebrate the refreshing goodness of cake on special occasions — or just because, with an overview of baking as a science and how that specifically applies to cake.

Enjoy the pleasures of candy without wrecking your diet. Some of these are remakes of classic recipes that bring your childhood flooding back, while a few may be a completely new experience.

Revel in the joy that pie brings throughout the year. One of the trickiest aspects of low-carb pies is finding an effective replacement for the crust, so you discover some white flour alternatives and how to use them.

Appreciate cookies that taste just like you remember grandma's and how you can maximize taste.

Value the cold sweetness of ice cream and frozen treats on a hot day. If you thought that these types of desserts went away when you adopted keto, you'll be happy to discover a variety of recipes that can bring back these refreshing sweet treats.

Relish the sweet simplicity of mug cakes and dump cakes without having to make a full cake.

Savor the pure, refreshing joy of milkshakes and smoothies, which you can consume whenever you have the urge.

Sip on a hot drink to warm the soul, whether you're starting your day in the cold midst of winter or settling down after a stressful day.

Start your efforts to drinking alcohol correctly while on keto, focusing on a variety of low-carb liquors and alternate ingredients.

Chapter 4

Baking Keto Cakes — Moist and Delicious

You may long for a perfect slice of cake. You may wish you could have cake and not have to worry about the carbs inside it. Well, with these fantastic recipes in this chapter, you definitely can. All these cake recipes are low-carb, made with healthy sweeteners, and never use white flours. Not only do they stick to the keto diet, but they are also delicious, and many of them are loaded with nutrients (like lots of healthy nuts).

Creating Classic Cakes, Keto Style

Many cakes out there are considered to be classics. A good chocolate cake recipe, for example, is something that every baker should have on hand. Luckily, we have re-created many classic types of cakes to fit into the keto diet, including a light lemon cake and New York cheesecake.

Making a classic cake keto-friendly doesn't have to be hard either. We have tried and tested each recipe to ensure that it encapsulated the essence of the original cake (moist, sweet, and irresistible!) while using only keto ingredients. You'll be pleasantly surprised when you love these keto cakes even more than their classic counterparts.

BAKING AS A SCIENCE

When you cook a meal, you often can adjust the recipe to suit your preferences. You can add a little extra salt at the end to bring out the flavor, or you can skip the chopped onion in the recipe if you don't have one on hand. Baking is much different, though; you need to measure correctly and follow the recipe exactly. If not, the baked good may not come out the way you wanted. This principle is especially true in keto cake baking. Each ingredient plays a crucial role in making a perfect cake.

- **Flour:** The flour you use is the primary structure builder of the cake, no matter you use almond flour, coconut flour, or any other type of keto flour. It's the main ingredient and binds the cake, creates the fluffy texture, and provides the most nutrients.

- **Sweetener:** Sweeteners not only add that delicious taste you're looking for in a cake recipe, but they also help soften it. Most sweeteners hold moisture, keeping the cake moist for several days after baking.

- **Eggs:** Eggs give the cake structure as well as flavor, moisture, and color. When eggs bake inside a cake, the proteins they carry coagulate and firm, allowing the cake to hold its shape after it's baked. Eggs can also act as a leaven agent when they're whipped before being added to a batter. The air mixed into the egg expands when cooking, puffing the cake up while the eggs set.

- **Fats:** Having fat in a cake is essential and fulfills several roles. First, the fat tenderizes the cake, making it moist and creating a smooth texture in your mouth. When the fat is creamed into the recipe (such as when you cream butter), you trap air inside the fluffy mix, which then acts as a leavening agent for the cake as well. Fat also adds lots of flavor, making the cake rich and tender.

- **Milk:** Milk adds richness and structure. Additionally, it can help the cake reach that perfect golden-brown color you're seeking. Milk adds flavor and moisture, preventing your cake from being too dry.

- **Flavorings:** Adding a flavoring agent such as vanilla extract can make a massive difference in taste. Even half a teaspoon of vanilla has a noticeable impact, sweetening the cake and enhancing the other flavors without adding any extra sugars.

Be sure to follow the instructions and quantities in the recipes to ensure you get the ideal low-carb cake that you've been dreaming about.

Lemon Chiffon Cake

INGREDIENTS

2 cups finely ground almond flour

½ cup coconut flour

¼ teaspoon sea salt

1 teaspoon baking soda

1 teaspoon baking powder

4 eggs, room temperature

⅔ cup granular erythritol

⅔ cup butter, melted and cooled

1½ teaspoon lemon extract

½ teaspoon vanilla extract

¼ cup lemon juice

1 tablespoon lemon zest

½ cup unsweetened coconut milk, canned

DIRECTIONS

1 Preheat your oven to 350 degrees F and prepare two 8-inch cake pans by greasing them thoroughly with butter.

2 Combine the almond flour, coconut flour, sea salt, baking soda, and baking powder in a large bowl and whisk together. Set aside.

3 In a separate bowl, combine the eggs, erythritol, melted butter, both extracts, lemon juice, and the lemon zest. Whisk together well. Add the coconut milk to the wet ingredients and whisk again. Add the dry ingredients to the wet mixture slowly, adding only about ½ cup at a time and whisking well after each addition to ensure everything is well blended and no lumps form.

4 Divide the batter between the two cake pans and place in the preheated oven to bake for 30 minutes or until a toothpick comes out of the center of the cake cleanly. Allow the cakes to cool completely and then remove from the cake pans and assemble using your favorite icing. Decorate and enjoy.

PER SERVING: *Calories 162; Fat 14g; Cholesterol 72mg; Sodium 203mg; Carbohydrates 15g (Dietary Fiber 2g, Sugar Alcohol 11g); Net Carbohydrates 2.6g; Protein 7g.*

NOTE: In addition to the toothpick test in Step 4, you'll know the cakes are finished baking when the tops of the cakes are golden brown.

🍅 Citrus Olive Oil Cake

PREP TIME: 10 MIN | COOK TIME: 30 MIN | YIELD: 8 SERVINGS

INGREDIENTS

2 cups almond flour

1 teaspoon baking powder

½ teaspoon baking soda

½ teaspoon salt

4 eggs

½ cup erythritol

¼ cup olive oil

½ teaspoon orange extract

1 teaspoon lemon zest

½ teaspoon lime zest

DIRECTIONS

1 Preheat your oven to 325 degrees F. Grease a 9-inch cake pan with butter and set aside.

2 Combine the almond flour, baking powder, baking soda, and salt together in a large bowl. In a separate bowl, whisk together the eggs, erythritol, olive oil, orange extract, and lemon and lime zests. Combine the wet and dry ingredients and whisk until a smooth batter forms.

3 Pour the batter into the cake pan and then bake for 30 minutes in the preheated oven. The cake will be golden brown, and the center of the cake will spring back when touched. Let the cake cool in the cake pan before removing it from the pan. Slice and enjoy.

PER SERVING: *Calories 262; Fat 23g; Cholesterol 106mg; Sodium 285mg; Carbohydrates 18g (Dietary Fiber 3g, Sugar Alcohol 12g); Net Carbohydrates 2.8g; Protein 9g.*

Strawberry Almond Cake

PREP TIME: 20 MIN	COOK TIME: 30 MIN	YIELD: 8 SERVINGS

INGREDIENTS

1 tablespoon granular erythritol

4 eggs, separated

½ cup granular erythritol

1 teaspoon vanilla extract

½ teaspoon almond extract

1 teaspoon baking powder

¼ teaspoon salt

1½ cups finely ground, blanched almond flour

1 cup diced strawberries

DIRECTIONS

1 Preheat your oven to 325 degrees F. Grease an 8-inch cake pan with butter and then sprinkle 1 tablespoon of granular erythritol in the pan and shake the pan to coat the bottom and sides of the pan with the sweetener.

2 Place the egg yolks and ¼ cup of the granular erythritol in a mixer fitted with a whisk attachment and whip until fluffy. Add the vanilla extract and almond extract and mix to combine. Set the mix aside for now.

3 In a separate bowl, whip the egg whites with the remaining erythritol until stiff peaks form. Set aside as well. Combine baking powder, salt, and almond flour in a bowl and then stir into the egg yolk mixture to make a thick batter.

4 Gently fold the whipped egg whites into the yolk mix carefully to keep the egg whites nice and fluffy. Fold in the strawberries and then pour the batter into the prepared pan.

5 Bake the cake for 30 minutes or until it's golden brown and a toothpick comes out cleanly from the center. Take the cake out of the oven and run a spatula around the edge of the pan to loosen the cake from the sides. Let cool completely before removing from the cake pan. Garnish with extra strawberries or sugar-free whipped cream.

PER SERVING: *Calories 87; Fat 6g; Cholesterol 106mg; Sodium 143mg; Carbohydrates 17g (Dietary Fiber 1g, Sugar Alcohol 13g); Net Carbohydrates 2.2g; Protein 5g.*

NOTE: Shaking the greased pan sprinkled with granular erythritol helps the cake batter cling to the pan and rise nicely.

🍅 New York Cheesecake

| PREP TIME: 15 MIN | COOK TIME: 90 MIN | YIELD: 12 SERVINGS |

INGREDIENTS

1½ cups cream cheese, room temperature

¼ cup butter, room temperature

1 cup powdered erythritol

3 eggs, room temperature

¾ cup sour cream

½ tablespoon vanilla extract

DIRECTIONS

1 Preheat your oven to 300 degrees F. Grease a 9-inch, spring-form cake pan and place a round piece of parchment in the bottom. Wrap the outside of the pan with aluminum foil and then set the pan aside.

2 Beat the cream cheese and butter together until light and fluffy in a medium bowl. Add the powdered erythritol to the bowl and beat to combine well. Add the eggs one at a time, scraping down the sides of the bowl after each one. Add the sour cream and vanilla extract and stir until a smooth batter forms. Pour the batter into the prepared pan and then place the pan in a water bath.

3 Bake in the preheated oven for about 50 minutes. After 45 minutes, start checking to see if the cheesecake has already set (the center should jiggle slightly but be firm around the edges).

4 Remove the cheesecake from the oven and let cool to room temperature. Then set in the fridge and let the cheesecake cool completely and then run a knife or spatula around the edge of the pan and remove the cake. Slice and serve.

PER SERVING: *Calories 114; Fat 11g; Cholesterol 81mg; Sodium 60mg; Carbohydrates 17g (Dietary Fiber 0g, Sugar Alcohol 16g); Net Carbohydrates 1g; Protein 2.5g.*

NOTE: Top the cheesecake with some homemade whipped cream, a few fresh or frozen berries, or a drizzle of unsweetened chocolate.

Butter Cake

INGREDIENTS

2 cups almond flour, blanched and finely ground

½ cup sour cream, room temperature

8 tablespoons butter, melted

3 eggs, room temperature

⅔ cup granular erythritol

1 teaspoon vanilla extract

1 teaspoon baking powder

4 tablespoons butter

⅓ cup granular erythritol

3 teaspoon vanilla extract

2 tablespoons water

DIRECTIONS

1 Preheat your oven to 350 degrees F. Grease a Bundt pan and set aside.

2 In a large mixing bowl, whisk together the almond flour, sour cream, melted butter, eggs, ⅔ cup erythritol, 1 teaspoon vanilla extract, and baking powder. Whisk until the batter is smooth. Pour the batter into the prepared Bundt pan and bake in the preheated oven for 30 minutes or until golden brown.

3 While the cake is baking, add 4 tablespoons butter, granular erythritol, and vanilla extract to a small sauce pan along with water. Bring the mixture to a boil, stirring to dissolve the erythritol. Remove from the heat and set aside.

4 Remove the baked cake from the oven and poke holes in the bottom of the cake using a knife or skewer. Pour the butter mixture from the saucepan over the cake, letting it soak into the holes. Allow the cake to cool completely in the pan before flipping it out and enjoying.

PER SERVING: *Calories 252; Fat 24g; Cholesterol 89mg; Sodium 54mg; Carbohydrates 20g (Dietary Fiber 2g, Sugar Alcohol 16g); Net Carbohydrates 2.3g; Protein 6g.*

🥥 Coconut Cake

INGREDIENTS

5 eggs, room temperature, separated

½ cup coconut flour

¼ cup granular erythritol

½ teaspoon sea salt

½ teaspoon xanthan gum

¼ cup butter, melted

¼ cup coconut oil, melted

1 teaspoon vanilla extract

8 ounces cream cheese, softened

¼ cup powdered erythritol

1 teaspoon vanilla extract

½ cup toasted shredded coconut, unsweetened

DIRECTIONS

1 Preheat your oven to 350 degrees F. Grease a loaf pan with butter and set aside.

2 Place the egg whites in a medium bowl and whip until stiff peaks form. Set aside. Add the coconut flour, granular erythritol, sea salt, and xanthan gum to a separate medium bowl and whisk together. Add the egg yolks, melted butter, coconut oil, and vanilla extract to the flour mix and stir together until a smooth batter forms. Fold the whipped egg whites into the batter gently and then pour the batter into the prepared pan.

3 Bake for 45 minutes or until the cake is golden brown.

4 While the cake is baking, make the frosting by whipping the cream cheese and powdered erythritol together until light and fluffy using an electric hand mixer. Add the vanilla extract and stir to combine.

5 After the cake has cooled, remove it from the pan and spread the frosting across the top. Sprinkle with the toasted coconut, slice, and serve.

PER SERVING: *Calories 256; Fat 24g; Cholesterol 143mg; Sodium 234mg; Carbohydrates 15g (Dietary Fiber 3g, Sugar Alcohol 9g); Net Carbohydrates 2.9g; Protein 6g.*

Pistachio Pound Cake

PREP TIME: 15 MIN	COOK TIME: 30 MIN	YIELD: 10 SERVINGS

INGREDIENTS

½ cup lemon juice

½ cup granular erythritol

3 eggs, room temperature

1 cup finely ground pistachios

2 cups finely ground almond flour

½ teaspoon baking soda

1 teaspoon vanilla extract

2 tablespoons coconut oil

1 tablespoon granular erythritol

½ teaspoon lemon extract

2 tablespoons water

½ cup chopped pistachios

DIRECTIONS

1 Preheat your oven to 350 degrees F. Grease a 9-inch springform pan.

2 In a large bowl, whisk together the lemon juice, ½ cup granular erythritol, eggs, pistachios, almond flour, baking soda, and vanilla extract. Whisk until a smooth batter forms. Pour the batter into the prepared pan and bake for about 30 minutes or until a toothpick comes out cleanly when inserted into the center of the cake.

3 While the cake is baking, combine the coconut oil, granular erythritol, lemon extract, and water in a small saucepan. Bring to a boil, stirring to dissolve the erythritol. Remove from the heat and set aside.

4 Remove the cooked cake from the oven and pour the glaze over the cake while it's still in the cake pan. Sprinkle the cake with the pistachios and then let the cake cool before removing the springform sides of the pan, slicing, and serving.

PER SERVING: Calories 266; Fat 22g; Cholesterol 64mg; Sodium 113mg; Carbohydrates 20g (Dietary Fiber 4g, Sugar Alcohol 11g); Net Carbohydrates 5.6g; Protein 10g.

Making Chocolate Cakes Keto

Following a keto diet means that a lot of chocolate you find in the grocery store is off-limits. You may be surprised to find that even the most basic, simple chocolate bars have added sugars, especially milk chocolate and white chocolate that not only tend to have sugar blended in but also various forms of milk that add carbohydrates.

Fortunately, you still have a lot of options when it comes to chocolate and keto baking. The first ingredient that is perfect for both the diet and to bake with is unsweetened cocoa powder. It's easy to find, has no sugar added, and will give your baked goods the deep, chocolatey taste that you may be craving.

You can also look for chocolate that has been specially made for keto baking. Many brands have created chocolate chips and chocolate baking ingredients using stevia and erythritol, so they don't have any added carbs and the chocolate is sweet. This section gives you some fantastic chocolate cake recipes that are completely keto-approved and also taste amazing. You're sure to find your new favorite chocolate dessert here.

IMPORTANT TRICKS TO BAKING A PERFECT KETO CAKE

Here are a few tips that can help you bake the perfect keto cake. Keep them in mind with every recipe you try, and you'll find that baking a beautiful cake is quite simple:

- **Make sure all your ingredients are room temperature when you begin.** Butter, eggs, milk, and every other component come together easily when they're the same temperature.

- **Scrape the mixing bowl well after each ingredient addition.** Sometimes ingredients tend to stick to the edges, which can prevent your batter and cake from turning out perfectly. Use a rubber spatula to scrape the bowl frequently.

- **Measure everything carefully.** Not measuring ingredients correctly is one of the biggest mistakes you can make in cake baking. Be sure to level every cup, teaspoon, and tablespoon accurately to ensure you add the correct quantity of ingredients.

- **Be careful when you begin considering ingredient substitutes because each recipe is written to use the specified item.** When you start replacing certain fats, flours, or liquids, the result will be a different cake. Try to stick to the ingredients in the recipe the first few times you make it. After you've mastered the core recipe, you can begin experimenting with replacements.

- **Place a piece of parchment paper in the bottom of the cake pan to make removing the cake from the pan easier.** Doing so makes the cake pop right out. Always grease baking pans well with butter or baking spray, use a parchment circle, and you'll never have a cake stuck in the pan again.

Chocolate Cake with Chocolate Whipped Cream

PREP TIME: 10 MIN	COOK TIME: 20 MIN	YIELD: 8 SERVINGS

INGREDIENTS

1½ cups almond flour

½ cup coconut flour

1 cup monk fruit erythritol blend

½ teaspoon sea salt

1 teaspoon baking powder

½ cup cocoa powder, unsweetened

¼ cup butter, melted

¼ cup coconut oil, melted

2 eggs

1½ teaspoons vanilla extract

1 cup coconut milk, unsweetened, canned

1 cup heavy whipping cream

1 teaspoon vanilla extract

1 teaspoon monk fruit erythritol blend

2 tablespoons cocoa powder, unsweetened

DIRECTIONS

1 Preheat your oven to 350 degrees F and grease two 8-inch cake pans with butter.

2 In a large mixing bowl, stir together the almond flour, coconut flour, 1 cup monk fruit erythritol, sea salt, baking powder, and cocoa powder. Add the melted butter, melted coconut oil, eggs, and vanilla extract to the dry ingredients and stir well until a smooth batter forms. Add the coconut milk to the batter and whisk to combine.

3 Divide the cake batter between the two prepared baking pans and then place the pans side by side in the preheated oven for 20 minutes or until a toothpick comes out of the center cleanly. Let the cakes cool completely and then remove from the cake pans. Place in the fridge until you're ready to frost and eat.

4 To make the chocolate whipped cream, add the heavy whipping cream, vanilla extract, monk fruit erythritol, and cocoa powder to a bowl or mixer fitted with a whisk attachment. Whip until stiff peaks form. Spread the chocolate whipped cream on the cooled cake, putting a thin layer over the entire top of one cake and then placing the second cake on top to stack it. Decorate as desired, using the whipped cream. Enjoy.

PER SERVING: *Calories 419; Fat 42g; Cholesterol 109mg; Sodium 205mg; Carbohydrates 32g (Dietary Fiber 3g, Sugar Alcohol 25g); Net Carbohydrates 4.3g; Protein 8g.*

Chocolate Pound Cake with Bacon Bourbon Frosting

PREP TIME: 15 MIN	COOK TIME: 60 MIN	YIELD: 12 SERVINGS

INGREDIENTS

½ cup butter, softened

2¼ cups granular erythritol

8 ounces cream cheese, softened

8 eggs, room temperature

1 teaspoon vanilla extract

1½ cups almond flour

½ cup cocoa powder, unsweetened

1 tablespoon baking powder

½ teaspoon kosher salt

2 ounces dark chocolate, unsweetened, melted

4 tablespoons butter, softened

¼ cup cream cheese, softened

2 tablespoons powdered erythritol

1 tablespoon bourbon

½ teaspoon bourbon vanilla extract

½ cup bacon, cooked and crumbled

DIRECTIONS

1 Preheat your oven to 325 degrees F. Grease a loaf pan with butter and set aside.

2 Beat the butter and granular erythritol until light and fluffy in the bowl of a stand mixer or a medium bowl with an electric hand mixer. Add the softened cream cheese and beat to combine. Add the eggs one at a time, scraping down the sides of the bowl after each addition to ensure everything is mixed evenly. Add the vanilla extract and blend into the batter. Add the almond flour, cocoa powder, baking powder, and salt and mix until the batter is smooth. Add the melted dark chocolate and beat well to incorporate fully. Pour the batter into the prepared loaf pan.

3 Bake for 60 minutes or until a toothpick comes out cleanly from the cake's center. Cool the cake completely before removing from the pan.

4 To make the frosting, place the butter, cream cheese, and powdered erythritol in a medium bowl and beat until fluffy. Add the bourbon and vanilla extract and mix well. Spread the frosting over the cooled pound cake and then sprinkle with the bacon. Slice and serve.

PER SERVING: *Calories 359; Fat 33g; Cholesterol 201mg; Sodium 356mg; Carbohydrates 15g (Dietary Fiber 4g, Sugar Alcohol 7g); Net Carbohydrates 4.2g; Protein 11g.*

Chapter **5**

Going Sweet with Keto Candies

When you think of candy, you may automatically think of sugar. And when you think about sugar, you may immediately decide that the candy isn't keto-approved. Although candy does revolve around sweetness, it doesn't have to come from processed high-carb sugar. You can use many amazing keto sweetener options when making candy so you can enjoy these great treats. Sugar isn't a requirement for enjoying candy, and in this chapter, we show you why in several delicious recipes.

Making Caramels and Fudge Candies

Caramel is traditionally made by cooking sugar until it's a golden brown and then adding cream or milk to create a caramel in the texture that you desire. Of course, granular sugar is off-limits to keto followers, but you can use other sugar alternatives to make caramel candies.

To cook caramels, you'll often need a candy thermometer in order to get the mixture to the correct temperature, ensuring that the caramel candy is the correct consistency. Although these candies may take a little bit to master, you'll be happy when you have perfected them, giving you a tasty keto caramel you can make and enjoy anytime.

In addition, fudge can be another classic candy that you can make keto-approved with the right ingredient substitutions. This section gives you a few caramel and fudge recipes.

🥔 Pecan Turtles

PREP TIME: 40 MIN	COOK TIME: 20 MIN	YIELD: 40 CANDIES

INGREDIENTS

4 tablespoons butter

1 cup heavy whipping cream

¾ cup golden granular erythritol

¼ teaspoon sea salt

½ teaspoon liquid stevia

1½ teaspoons vanilla extract

2 cups toasted pecans, whole

½ cup sugar-free, dark chocolate chips

1 Place the butter in medium saucepan and heat on the stovetop over medium heat. Allow the butter to melt and start to brown. Add the heavy whipping cream, granular erythritol, and sea salt to the saucepan, whisking slowly and steadily. The mix will bubble immediately and then die down.

2 Lower the heat to low and cook the caramel for about 10 minutes or until the caramel reaches about 235 degrees F, letting it thicken and brown. Keep an eye on the caramel, ensuring it doesn't burn. Remove the caramel from the heat and add the stevia liquid and vanilla extract. Stir to combine well and then let the mix cool for about 5 minutes. Add the toasted pecans to the caramel mix and stir.

3 Scoop the caramel and pecan mix onto a parchment- or silicone-lined sheet tray, making small dollops that are about 1 teaspoon in size. You may need multiple sheet trays. Place the sheet trays in the fridge for 30 minutes to let the caramel firm.

4 Melt the dark chocolate over a double boiler, stirring until the chips are completely melted and smooth. Drizzle the melted chocolate over the chilled caramels. After the chocolate is firm, place the candies in an airtight container and enjoy. Store for about two weeks at room temperature. Store in the freezer for up to one month.

PER SERVING: *Calories 49; Fat 5g; Cholesterol 11mg; Sodium 15mg; Carbohydrates 5g (Dietary Fiber 1g, Sugar Alcohol 4g); Net Carbohydrates .5g; Protein .4g.*

NOTE: In Step 1, stir until the bubbles stop.

NOTE: In Step 2, the caramel should be a nice brown.

☕ Peanut Butter Fudge

INGREDIENTS

8 ounces cream cheese

½ pound butter

1 cup smooth peanut butter, unsweetened

1 teaspoon vanilla extract

¼ teaspoon sea salt

1 cup powdered erythritol

½ cup vanilla whey protein powder

DIRECTIONS

1 Grease a 9x9-inch pan with coconut oil and place a piece of parchment in the bottom. Set aside.

2 Add the cream cheese and butter to a small saucepan and heat over medium heat, stirring constantly to melt and combine the ingredients. Add the peanut butter to the pan and stir to melt and combine as well. Remove the pan from the heat and add the vanilla extract, sea salt, powdered erythritol, and protein powder. Stir well and then pour the mix into an electric stand mixer. Blend in the stand mixer until the mix begins to cool and is completely mixed together.

3 Pour the fudge into the greased pan and spread evenly. Place in the fridge to chill and set completely. Slice the fudge and enjoy or store in an airtight container in the fridge for up to one month.

PER SERVING: *Calories 114; Fat 11g; Cholesterol 21mg; Sodium 46mg; Carbohydrates 7g (Dietary Fiber 1g, Sugar Alcohol 5g); Net Carbohydrates 1.2g; Protein 2g.*

Chewy Caramels

PREP TIME: 10 MIN	COOK TIME: 20 MIN	YIELD: 16 PIECES

INGREDIENTS

¼ cup heavy whipping cream

1 tablespoon butter

1½ cups granular erythritol and monk fruit blend

¼ cup water

½ teaspoon vanilla extract

DIRECTIONS

1 Place the heavy whipping cream and butter in a microwave-safe dish and heat for one minute, allowing the butter to melt completely. Stir to blend and then set aside.

2 Place the granular erythritol and monk fruit blend in a small saucepan along with the water and vanilla extract. Heat the saucepan mix over medium heat. Use a candy thermometer to watch the temperature of the mix. Cook to 350 degrees F. When the color changes to a deep golden brown, remove the pan from the heat.

3 Whisk the butter and cream mix into the caramel slowly. Place the saucepan back over the heat and cook, whisking constantly until the mix browns more. It should be the color of dark caramel.

4 Pour the caramel onto a rimmed sheet tray lined with parchment or a silicone mat. Chill in the fridge until the caramel has set and cooled completely. Cut and wrap each caramel individually in small pieces of parchment paper. Store in the fridge for up to one month.

PER SERVING: *Calories 20; Fat 2g; Cholesterol 7mg; Sodium 2mg; Carbohydrates 6g (Dietary Fiber 0g, Sugar Alcohol 6g); Net Carbohydrates 0g; Protein .1g.*

NOTE: In Step 3, the mixture will bubble and steam but will subside as you stir.

Coconut Candies

INGREDIENTS

1½ cups heavy whipping cream

1½ tablespoons butter

¼ cup powdered erythritol

2 cups powdered erythritol

2 cups shredded, unsweetened coconut flakes

2 tablespoons coconut oil

12 ounces dark baking chocolate

DIRECTIONS

1 Line a sheet tray with parchment paper and set aside.

2 Place the heavy whipping cream, butter, and ¼ cup powdered erythritol in a small sauce pan and bring to a boil. Reduce the heat to a simmer and cook until reduced by half, which should take about 10 minutes. Stir frequently.

3 Combine the remaining 2 cups powdered erythritol, coconut flakes, and thickened heavy whipping cream mix in a large bowl. Mix well and then scoop into small, ½ tablespoon–sized balls, placing them on the prepared sheet tray. Refrigerate the coconut balls for about 30 minutes or until nice and firm.

4 Place the coconut oil and dark chocolate in a double boiler and melt over medium heat, stirring occasionally until smooth. Dip the chilled coconut balls in the chocolate, submerging them completely and then returning them to the sheet tray.

5 After all the coconut centers are dipped, return the tray to the fridge to keep them cool. Store in an airtight container and keep refrigerated for up to one month.

PER SERVING: *Calories 122; Fat 12g; Cholesterol 17mg; Sodium 6mg; Carbohydrates 22g (Dietary Fiber 4g, Sugar Alcohol 16g); Net Carbohydrates 2.5g; Protein 1g.*

Trying Some Tasty and Quick Keto Candies

Making candy isn't always a long process. In fact, the following candy recipes create delicious keto-approved candy recipes and some require very little to no cooking time at all. That means you can satisfy your candy craving quickly!

When deciding which candies to make and how much candy to make, consider the time it takes to cook the candies and also how to store them. Most of these candies will last a few days if not longer, so making a double (or triple) batch may be worth it.

AMAZING KETO SWEETENERS FOR CANDIES

Using a keto sweetener alternative can be tricky because many sugar alternatives don't behave the way sugar does. For example, white cane sugar caramelizes easily, making it perfect for a variety of candies. White cane sugar also dissolves completely when warmed and doesn't immediately burn when cooked. When you start to make candy using low-carb sweeteners, you need to select one that mimics the way sugar acts in the recipe you're using. We discuss many sweetener alternatives in Chapter 19. Here are a few of our favorites that achieve the same texture and taste as a candy made with regular white sugar:

- **Erythritol:** Erythritol is pulled from the food source and then mixed with water and dried to form a crystal that's similar to white cane sugar. It melts when heated in much the same manner as sugar, so it's perfect for candy making.

- **Stevia**: Stevia typically has a finer consistency than cane sugar, and you need much less of it in a recipe to get the correct sweetness level. You can also purchase liquid stevia, adding a nice sweet flavor to candy with just one or two drops.

- **Monk fruit:** Monk fruit is much sweeter than cane sugar and is often blended with dextrose or erythritol to balance out the sweetness. There are almost no adverse side effects to consuming monk fruit, and it has zero carbs or calories. This sweetener comes in liquid, granule, and also powdered forms and is excellent for candy making!

Peppermint Bark

| PREP TIME: 10 MIN | COOK TIME: 5 MIN | YIELD: 8 CANDIES |

INGREDIENTS

9 ounces baking chocolate

14 sugar-free peppermint candies, unwrapped

½ teaspoon peppermint extract

DIRECTIONS

1 Place the chocolate in a bowl over a double boiler and melt, stirring occasionally, over medium-low heat.

2 While the chocolate is melting, crush the peppermint candies by pulsing them in a food processor or smashing them with a rolling pin. Set about 2 tablespoons of the crushed candies aside and then add the remaining crushed peppermint to the melted chocolate along with the peppermint extract. Stir together. Pour the melted chocolate mix onto a sheet tray with a silicone baking mat or piece of parchment paper and spread into a thin layer. Sprinkle the reserved crushed peppermint over the top of the chocolate.

3 Let the chocolate cool until firm and then break into pieces. Store in an airtight container in the fridge for up to one month.

PER SERVING: Calories 131; Fat 10g; Cholesterol 0mg; Sodium 0mg; Carbohydrates 29g (Dietary Fiber 9g, Sugar Alcohol 15g); Net Carbohydrates 4.6g; Protein 2g.

FINDING TOOLS FOR MAKING CANDY

You need to consider purchasing a few essential tools that can help you make perfect candies. They are as follows:

- **Candy thermometer:** This tool is an ideal place to start. Many sweets require you to cook the sugar or other ingredients to a specific temperature, and a good candy thermometer helps you do just that.

- **Silicone baking mat:** A quality silicone baking mat is also quite helpful. These mats can withstand high temperatures and don't stick to the candy after it cools.

- **Candy molds:** Molds are a good idea to have on hand to consistently make nice, uniform keto candy.

The more candy you make, the more useful you'll find each of these tools. You'll be happy that you have them on hand when you want to make yourself a keto treat.

Sea Salt Almond Bark

PREP TIME: 10 MIN | COOK TIME: 15 MIN | YIELD: 20 PIECES

INGREDIENTS

½ cup granular erythritol

4 tablespoons water

1 tablespoon butter

1½ cups almonds, toasted, whole

½ teaspoon sea salt

½ cup cocoa butter

⅓ cup dark chocolate chips, unsweetened

½ cup powdered erythritol

¾ cup cocoa powder, unsweetened

½ teaspoon vanilla extract

DIRECTIONS

1   Prepare a sheet tray by lining it with parchment paper or a silicone mat.

2   Add the granular erythritol and 4 tablespoons of water in a small saucepan and heat over medium heat. Bring to a boil and cook for about 4 minutes to darken. Remove the pan from the heat, let cool for 1 minute and then add the butter, whisking to combine it well. Add the almonds to the pot and stir to completely coat them in the caramel. Stir in the sea salt and then pour the mix onto the prepared sheet tray. Set aside.

3   In a clean small saucepan, melt the cocoa butter over low heat and then add the chocolate chips. Stir until smooth. Add the powdered erythritol and cocoa powder and stir until smooth. Turn off the heat and add the vanilla extract to the chocolate mix. Pour the chocolate over the caramelized almonds and spread to cover the nuts completely in the chocolate.

4   Sprinkle some extra sea salt over the chocolate and then set aside to cool. Once the chocolate bark is firm, break into pieces and store in an airtight container.

PER SERVING: *Calories 87; Fat 9g; Cholesterol 2mg; Sodium 51mg; Carbohydrates 14g (Dietary Fiber 2g, Sugar Alcohol 10g); Net Carbohydrates 1.7g; Protein 1g.*

NOTE: When bringing the granulated erythritol to boil, it may smoke slightly, but that's okay.

Coffee Gummies

PREP TIME: 15 MIN	COOK TIME: 5 MIN	YIELD: 10 SERVINGS OR 80 MINI GUMMY BEARS

INGREDIENTS

4 tablespoons unflavored gelatin powder

15 grams instant coffee powder

¾ cup water

3 tablespoons heavy whipping cream

10 drops chocolate liquid stevia

DIRECTIONS

1 Add the gelatin and water to a small saucepan. Let sit for 5 minutes to bloom the gelatin and then place all the remaining ingredients into a small saucepan. Heat over medium heat, whisking constantly until the mix is smooth and everything is completely melted.

2 Remove the pan from the heat and use a dropper to divide the mix into a gummy bear mold.

3 Place the gummy bears in the fridge to chill for at least two hours. Pop the gummy bears out of the mold and store in an airtight container in the fridge for up to one month.

PER SERVING: *Calories 30; Fat 2g; Cholesterol 6mg; Sodium 8mg; Carbohydrates 1.6g (Dietary Fiber 0g, Sugar Alcohol 0g); Net Carbohydrates 1.6g; Protein 2.6g.*

Strawberry Fat Bombs

PREP TIME: 1 HOUR PLUS 10 MIN	COOK TIME: 0 MIN	YIELD: 24 PIECES

INGREDIENTS

1½ cups fresh, chopped strawberries

1 teaspoon vanilla extract

½ pound cream cheese, room temperature

1 stick butter, room temperature

¼ cup powdered erythritol

DIRECTIONS

1 Place the strawberries and vanilla extract in a food processor and puree until smooth. Add the cream cheese and butter to the food processor and blend until well combined. Add the powdered erythritol and blend again, ensuring everything is combined completely.

2 Scoop the mix into a greased mini muffin tray. Place in a freezer to chill for at least 1 hour.

3 After firm, remove from the muffin tray and place in an airtight container to store. Keep in the freezer for up to three months.

PER SERVING: *Calories 70; Fat 7g; Cholesterol 21mg; Sodium 35mg; Carbohydrates 3g (Dietary Fiber 0g, Sugar Alcohol 2g); Net Carbohydrates 1g; Protein 1g.*

NOTE: You can use any shaped, small silicone molds. A silicone ice tray works as well.

🍓 Peanut Butter and Jelly Cups

PREP TIME: 3 HOURS	COOK TIME: 15 MIN	YIELD: 12 CANDIES

INGREDIENTS

½ cup unsalted peanuts

1 tablespoon coconut oil (firm)

2 tablespoons cashew butter

1 tablespoon granular erythritol

1 tablespoon coconut flour

1 cup fresh chopped strawberries

4 drops liquid stevia

¾ cup finely chopped unsweetened chocolate

DIRECTIONS

1 Place 12 mini paper muffin liners in a mini muffin tray. Put the peanuts, coconut oil, cashew butter, granular erythritol, and coconut flour in a food processor and pulse until the mix is well combined until it's a thick paste.

2 Scoop the mix into the 12 paper muffin cups, dividing the mix evenly. Press the peanut butter mix into the paper liners, compacting as much as possible, and then place the tray in the freezer until the mix is frozen solid, about 1 hour.

3 Add the strawberries and liquid stevia to the food processor and puree until smooth. Take the muffin tray out of the freezer and scoop the strawberry jelly mix over the peanut butter layer. Return the tray to the freezer for another 2 hours.

4 Melt the chocolate over a double boiler, stirring until smooth. Take the muffin tray out of the freezer and pour the melted chocolate over the jelly layer, filling the mini muffin cup to the top with chocolate.

5 Return the tray to the freezer one more time and allow the candies to firm completely, about 20 minutes. Store in the freezer until you're ready to enjoy. Remove the paper liner and eat.

PER SERVING: *Calories 82; Fat 7g; Cholesterol 0mg; Sodium 1mg; Carbohydrates 10g (Dietary Fiber 4g, Sugar Alcohol 3g); Net Carbohydrates 3.3g; Protein 2g.*

NOTE: In Step 1, pulse the mix until you have a thick paste.

Chapter **6**

Enjoying Keto Pies and Tarts

Pie may be one dessert that you crave but are hesitant to make. After all, a traditional pie does contain a lot of carbs, so you may ask how can you possibly make it keto-friendly?! Fortunately, we include a number of fantastic low-carb pie recipes in this chapter that are easy to make and taste delicious. These range from fruit pies to decadent chocolate creations and all of them can fit into your macros.

Baking Perfect Pies

The idea of a fresh pie baking in the oven is something that makes almost anyone excited for dessert. In fact, one of the best smells in the world is that of a freshly baked pie — it just makes a home seem welcoming and shows how much love you have put into baking. These keto pies in this section give you all of those feelings and more.

We have perfected keto pie crusts, giving you a few different crusts that you can enjoy. Although our pie fillings are also amazing, keep the crust recipes in mind and fill them with any keto-friendly filling you want. There are many ways to bake a perfect pie and low-carb restrictions won't stop you from enjoying a fresh, oven-baked tradition.

🍅 Chocolate Cream Pie

PREP TIME: 15 MIN	COOK TIME: 25 MIN	YIELD: 10 SERVINGS

INGREDIENTS

2 cups almond flour

½ teaspoon sea salt

2 tablespoons granular erythritol

2 tablespoons coconut oil

1 tablespoon gelatin

¼ cup warm water

2 tablespoons boiling water

One 15-ounce can unsweetened coconut cream

3 egg yolks

½ cup granular erythritol

½ tablespoon xanthan gum

¼ cup finely chopped baking chocolate

¼ teaspoon vanilla extract

One 15-ounce can unsweetened coconut cream

1 teaspoon gelatin

2 tablespoons warm water

2 tablespoons powdered erythritol

1 teaspoon vanilla extract

¼ teaspoon sea salt

DIRECTIONS

1 Preheat your oven to 350 degrees F.

2 Make the pie crust by placing the almond flour, ½ teaspoon sea salt, 2 tablespoons granular erythritol, and coconut oil in a food processor. In a separate small bowl combine the 1 tablespoon of gelatin with ¼ cup warm water and let sit to bloom for 5 minutes. Add 2 tablespoons boiling water to the gelatin and whisk to melt. Pour the hot liquid gelatin mix into the food processor and pulse until a smooth dough forms.

3 Remove the dough and place on a silicone baking mat. Place a piece of parchment paper over the top of the dough and use a rolling pin to flatten the dough, rolling it between the parchment and the silicone mat. Then flip the dough into a 9-inch pie pan. Bake the crust in the preheated oven for about 15 minutes or until it has turned a nice golden brown.

4 Make the chocolate filling by placing the coconut cream in a small saucepan. Heat over medium heat until slightly simmering. Place the egg yolks in a medium bowl and whisk. Slowly whisk in the hot coconut milk. Pour the mixture back into the sauce pan, add the ½ cup granular erythritol and xanthan gum. Heat the mixture over low heat, whisking constantly until it has thickened slightly. Remove from the heat and add the chocolate and vanilla extract. Whisk until the chocolate is melted and combined well.

5 Pour the chocolate mix into the baked pie crust and then place a piece of plastic wrap on top of the chocolate filling and move the pie to the fridge to cool completely.

(continued)

6 To make the cream topping, begin by placing the 1 teaspoon gelatin in a small bowl with 2 tablespoons warm water and let sit for 5 minutes. Microwave for 10 seconds to melt. Place can of coconut milk in a chilled mixing bowl and whip until fluffy. Add the melted gelatin, powdered erythritol, vanilla extract, and ¼ teaspoon sea salt and whip until soft peaks form. Spread the whipped cream over the top of the completely cooled chocolate pie. Slice and serve or store in the fridge for up to two days.

PER SERVING: *Calories 362; Fat 35g; Cholesterol 55mg; Sodium 185mg; Carbohydrates 24g (Dietary Fiber 4g, Sugar Alcohol 15g); Net Carbohydrates 5g; Protein 8g.*

SAYING GOODBYE TO WHITE FLOUR

The main ingredient in every single crust in pie recipes that aren't keto is likely to be all-purpose white flour. Even the crusts that involve cookies are graham crackers, which are based on white flour. As a keto dieter, you know that white flour is off-limits, but it's not something you can just eliminate — you also need to find a great keto replacement. To make perfect pies, you need to find a new flour to make a delicious pie crust, and the following are great options:

- **Almond flour:** Almond flour is fantastic for pie crusts. You can easily replace white flour in any pie crust recipe with an equal amount of finely ground almond flour. Almond flour contains many beneficial nutrients and healthy fats, making it an excellent addition to a low-carb diet. The flour also is nice and fluffy, which is perfect for a flaky pie crust. Pie crust can be a little dense when baking it (which is usually the texture of almond-flour-based baked goods). Almond flour is a pie's best friend.

- **Coconut flour:** Coconut flour, which is made by grinding the dried pulp of a coconut, works wonderfully in pie crust and has a subtle flavor. If you bake a crust with coconut flour, you probably won't taste the coconut at all, because the pie filling will easily overpower it. Coconut flour is incredibly absorbent, so you'll need to add additional liquid (eggs pair well here). Depending on the effect you're going for, you may want to consider using half the amount of coconut flour and replacing the other half with almond flour.

- **Sugar-free cookies:** Lots of pies use cookies or graham crackers mixed with melted butter to create a quick and easy crumbly crust. You can make keto cookie crumbs by crushing the cookies in a food processor until tiny crumbs form. Then, use these carb-free cookie crumbs as you would use graham cracker crumbs. Any kind of cookie will do, so feel free to use your favorite.

🍅 Lemon Curd Pie

| PREP TIME: 20 MIN | COOK TIME: 35 MIN | YIELD: 10 SERVINGS |

INGREDIENTS

2 cups almond flour

½ teaspoon sea salt

2 tablespoons powdered erythritol

2 tablespoons coconut oil

1 tablespoon gelatin

¼ cup warm water

2 tablespoons boiling water

1 cup coconut cream

4 egg yolks

½ cup lemon juice

1 tablespoon lemon zest

¼ cup butter

1 teaspoon vanilla extract

¼ teaspoon xanthan gum

½ cup powdered erythritol

1 cup sour cream

DIRECTIONS

1 Preheat your oven to 350 degrees F.

2 Make the pie crust by placing the almond flour, ½ teaspoon sea salt, 2 tablespoons powdered erythritol, and coconut oil in a food processor. In a separate small bowl combine the 1 tablespoon gelatin with ¼ cup warm water and let sit to bloom for 5 minutes. Add 2 tablespoons boiling water to the gelatin and whisk to melt. Pour the hot liquid gelatin mix into the food processor and pulse until a smooth dough forms.

3 Remove the dough and place on a silicone baking mat. Place a piece of parchment paper over the top of the dough and use a rolling pin to flatten the dough, rolling it between the parchment and the silicone mat. Remove the parchment from the top of the dough and then flip the dough into a 9-inch pie pan, peeling the silicone mat off the dough after it's in the pie pan. Bake the crust in the preheated oven for about 15 minutes or until it has turned a nice golden brown.

4 To make the filling, combine the coconut cream, egg yolks, lemon juice, and lemon zest in a large saucepan. Whisk the mix over medium heat until it begins to thicken. Remove the pan from the heat and add the butter and vanilla extract to the mix and stir well, letting the butter melt and blend in. Sprinkle the xanthan gum over the top of the mix and whisk in as well. Add the powdered erythritol and whisk again. Add the sour cream, whisking well to mix in completely and then pour the filling into the baked pie shell.

5 Place the pie in the fridge to cool completely and then serve with your favorite keto whipped cream or enjoy as is.

PER SERVING: *Calories 314; Fat 30g; Cholesterol 98mg; Sodium 124mg; Carbohydrates 19g (Dietary Fiber 2g, Sugar Alcohol 12g); Net Carbohydrates 4.4g; Protein 8g.*

🍓 Strawberry Cream Pie

PREP TIME: 20 MIN	COOK TIME: 15 MIN	YIELD: 10 SERVINGS

INGREDIENTS

2 cups almond flour

½ teaspoon sea salt

2 tablespoons powdered erythritol

2 tablespoons coconut oil

1 tablespoon gelatin

¼ cup warm water

2 tablespoons boiling water

1½ ounces freeze-dried strawberries

½ cup powdered erythritol

¼ teaspoon sea salt

1 cup plain Greek yogurt

1 tablespoon lemon juice

1 teaspoon vanilla extract

1 cup heavy whipping cream

DIRECTIONS

1 Preheat your oven to 350 degrees F.

2 Make the pie crust by placing the almond flour, ½ teaspoon sea salt, 2 tablespoons powdered erythritol, and coconut oil in a food processor. In a separate small bowl combine the 1 tablespoon of gelatin with ¼ cup warm water and let sit to bloom for 5 minutes. Add 2 tablespoons boiling water to the gelatin and whisk to melt. Pour the hot liquid gelatin mix into the food processor and pulse until a smooth dough forms.

3 Remove the dough and place on a silicone baking mat. Place a piece of parchment paper over the top of the dough and use a rolling pin to flatten the dough, rolling it between the parchment and the silicone mat. Remove the parchment from the top of the dough and then flip the dough into a 9-inch pie pan, peeling the silicone mat off the dough after it's in the pie pan. Bake the crust in the preheated oven for about 15 minutes or until it has turned a nice golden brown.

4 To make the filling, place the freeze-dried strawberries in a food processor and pulse until they're completely powdered. Add the powdered erythritol and sea salt and pulse again. Add the Greek yogurt, lemon juice, and vanilla extract to the food processor and mix until combined.

5 In a large bowl, whip the heavy whipping cream until stiff peaks form. Fold half of the whipped cream into the strawberry mix and then pour into the baked pie shell, smoothing evenly. Top the pie with the remaining whipped cream and serve. Store in the fridge for up to one day (best when enjoyed within the same day).

PER SERVING: *Calories 186; Fat 14g; Cholesterol 2mg; Sodium 162mg; Carbohydrates 21g (Dietary Fiber 2g, Sugar Alcohol 12g); Net Carbohydrates 6.3g; Protein 7g.*

French Silk Pie

PREP TIME: 2 HOURS 30 MIN

COOK TIME: 15 MIN

YIELD: 10 SERVINGS

INGREDIENTS

2 cups almond flour

½ teaspoon sea salt

2 tablespoons powdered erythritol

2 tablespoons coconut oil

1 tablespoon gelatin

¼ cup warm water

2 tablespoons boiling water

⅔ cup canned coconut milk, unsweetened, full fat

8 teaspoons unsweetened cocoa powder

5 tablespoons powdered erythritol

½ ripe avocado

¼ teaspoon vanilla extract

¼ teaspoon sea salt

1 cup heavy whipping cream

2 tablespoons powdered erythritol

DIRECTIONS

1 Preheat your oven to 350 degrees F.

2 Make the pie crust by placing the almond flour, ½ teaspoon sea salt, 2 tablespoons powdered erythritol, and coconut oil in a food processor. In a separate small bowl combine the 1 tablespoon of gelatin with ¼ cup warm water and let sit to bloom for 5 minutes. Add 2 tablespoons boiling water to the gelatin and whisk to melt. Pour the hot liquid gelatin mix into the food processor and pulse until a smooth dough forms.

3 Remove the dough and place on a silicone baking mat. Place a piece of parchment paper over the top of the dough and use a rolling pin to flatten the dough, rolling it between the parchment and the silicone mat. Remove the parchment from the top of the dough and then flip the dough into a 9-inch pie pan, peeling the silicone mat off the dough after it's in the pie pan. Bake the crust in the preheated oven for about 15 minutes or until it has turned a nice golden brown.

4 To make the filling, place all the ingredients into a large bowl. Blend together with an immersion blender until completely smooth. Pour the chocolate filling into the baked pie crust and place in the fridge for at least 2 hours to chill.

5 Whip the heavy whipping cream in a large bowl until stiff peaks form. Add the 2 tablespoons powdered erythritol and beat again. Spread the whipped cream over the chocolate cream pie and serve.

PER SERVING: *Calories 302; Fat 29g; Cholesterol 33mg; Sodium 164mg; Carbohydrates 18g (Dietary Fiber 4g, Sugar Alcohol 11g); Net Carbohydrates 3.5g; Protein 7g.*

Coconut Almond Tart

PREP TIME: 25 MIN	COOK TIME: 35 MIN	YIELD: 8 SERVINGS

INGREDIENTS

½ cup almond flour

¼ cup coconut flour

½ cup powdered erythritol

1 teaspoon vanilla extract

1 egg

2 tablespoons butter

3 eggs

½ cup granular erythritol

⅓ cup butter, melted

1 teaspoon almond extract

1 teaspoon vanilla extract

2 cups unsweetened, shredded coconut

DIRECTIONS

1 Place the almond flour, coconut flour, ½ cup powdered erythritol, 1 teaspoon vanilla extract, 1 egg, and 2 tablespoons butter in a food processor. Blend until a smooth dough forms. Roll the dough between two pieces of parchment until it is about 10 inches in diameter. Place in the fridge for about 30 minutes to cool.

2 While the dough is cooling, make the coconut filling. Begin by beating 3 eggs until light and fluffy. Add the ½ cup granular erythritol to the eggs and whip again. Pour in the melted butter and both extracts, blending until fully combined. Add the coconut and stir.

3 Preheat the oven to 375 degrees F.

4 Press the chilled dough into an 8-inch tart pan, pushing the dough up the sides of the pan and making the crust as even as possible. Pour the coconut mix into the dough and bake for 35 minutes. The top of the tart will be golden brown. Let cool completely before slicing and serving.

PER SERVING: *Calories 275; Fat 26g; Cholesterol 99mg; Sodium 35mg; Carbohydrates 31g (Dietary Fiber 3g, Sugar Alcohol 24g); Net Carbohydrates 3.7g; Protein 5g.*

Embracing No-Bake Pies

No-bake pie filling works wonderfully for keto pies because they're primarily cream based. This cream filling is set using gelatin or a baked egg yolk mixture. You can get a lot of flavor into this type of filling with very little effort. No-bake pies are incredibly versatile, enabling you to make a keto fruit-flavored pie, something chocolatey, or a delicious, nutty concoction. Many no-bake pies are frozen, creating the perfect warm-weather treat. No matter what kind of no-bake pie you make, having a dessert that is ready to eat without ever turning on the oven is simply amazing. These recipes are a few examples that require zero cooking time.

Peanut Butter Pie

PREP TIME: 20 MIN	COOK TIME: 0 MIN	YIELD: 12 SERVINGS

INGREDIENTS

4 cups walnuts

¼ cup butter, melted

2 tablespoons powdered erythritol

¼ teaspoon salt

½ teaspoon vanilla extract

2 tablespoons unsweetened cocoa powder

¾ cup unsweetened, smooth peanut butter

½ cup cream cheese

⅓ cup powdered erythritol

1 teaspoon vanilla extract

1¼ cups heavy whipping cream

DIRECTIONS

1 Place the walnuts in a food processor and pulse until they're fine crumbs. Add the butter and 2 tablespoons powdered erythritol, salt, vanilla extract, and cocoa powder to the food processor and pulse again until a dough forms. Place the crust mix into a pie tin and press into the bottom of the pan and up the sides. Place the pie crust in the freezer while you make the filling.

2 In the bowl of a stand mixer, beat the peanut butter, cream cheese, and ⅓ cup powdered erythritol until smooth and light. Add the vanilla extract and ¼ cup of the heavy whipping cream to the bowl and beat again until the filling has the consistency of frosting.

3 In a separate bowl, whip the remaining heavy whipping cream until stiff. Fold the heavy whipping cream together with the peanut butter mix and then transfer to the prepared pie crust, spreading the filling smooth.

4 Place the pie in the freezer for at least one hour. Slice and serve.

PER SERVING: *Calories 322; Fat 31g; Cholesterol 55mg; Sodium 107mg; Carbohydrates 13g (Dietary Fiber 2g, Sugar Alcohol 7g); Net Carbohydrates 4g; Protein 7g.*

🍫 Grasshopper Mousse Pie

PREP TIME: 20 MIN	COOK TIME: 10 MIN	YIELD: 12 SERVINGS

INGREDIENTS

4 cups walnuts

¼ cup butter, melted

2 tablespoons powdered erythritol

¼ teaspoon salt

½ teaspoon vanilla extract

2 tablespoons unsweetened cocoa powder

2½ cups heavy whipping cream

½ cup fresh mint, chopped

2 teaspoons gelatin

3 tablespoons warm water

4 egg yolks

½ cup powdered erythritol

½ teaspoon peppermint extract

DIRECTIONS

1 Place the walnuts in a food processor and pulse until they're fine crumbs. Add the butter and 2 tablespoons powdered erythritol, salt, vanilla extract, and cocoa powder to the food processor and pulse again until a dough forms. Place the crust mix into a pie tin and press into the bottom of the pan and up the sides. Place the pie crust in the freezer while you make the filling.

2 Place 1½ cups heavy whipping cream and the fresh mint in a small saucepan and bring to a boil. Turn off the heat, cover, and set aside to steep for 30 minutes. Strain the mint leaves from the cream, discarding them.

3 In a clean saucepan, combine the gelatin and warm water and let sit for 4 minutes to gel. Add the heavy whipping cream to the pot with the gelatin and whisk. Heat over medium heat, whisking constantly until the gelatin is fully dissolved.

4 In a medium bowl, whisk the yolks together with the powdered erythritol. Slowly whisk in the heavy whipping cream mixture and then transfer the yolk and cream mix back into the saucepan. Heat over low heat, whisking constantly, until the mixture reaches 160 degrees F on a candy thermometer. Remove from the heat, add the peppermint extract, cover, and refrigerate for about 1 hour. Whip the remaining heavy whipping cream in a large bowl until stiff peaks form.

5 Fold the whipped cream into the mint mix and then pour into the prepared pie crust. Spread evenly and serve while cool.

PER SERVING: *Calories 289; Fat 30g; Cholesterol 140mg; Sodium 65mg; Carbohydrates 14g (Dietary Fiber 1g, Sugar Alcohol 10g); Net Carbohydrates 2.6g; Protein 4g.*

☕ No-Bake Cheesecake Pie

PREP TIME: 3 HOURS	COOK TIME: 0 MIN	YIELD: 10 SERVINGS

INGREDIENTS

1½ cups finely ground almond flour

¼ cup powdered erythritol

¼ cup butter, melted

1½ cups cream cheese, softened

2 tablespoons sour cream

2 tablespoons lemon juice

¾ cups powdered erythritol

1 tablespoon gelatin

2 tablespoons warm water

½ cup heavy whipping cream

DIRECTIONS

1 Make the pie crust by mixing the almond flour, ¼ cup powdered erythritol, and melted butter together until crumbly. Press the mix into the bottom of a 9-inch pie pan and up the sides. Place in the fridge to firm.

2 To make the cheesecake filling, beat the cream cheese, sour cream, lemon juice, and ¾ cup powdered erythritol together until smooth. In a separate bowl, combine the gelatin with 2 tablespoons water and let sit for 1 minute. Microwave the mix for 25 seconds, melting the gelatin completely. Stir the melted gelatin into the cream cheese mix.

3 In a separate large bowl, whip the heavy whipping cream until stiff peaks form. Fold the whipped cream into the cream cheese mix and then spread the filling into the chilled pie crust.

4 Place in the fridge for at least 2 hours to firm. Slice and serve.

PER SERVING: *Calories 307; Fat 30g; Cholesterol 68mg; Sodium 135mg; Carbohydrates 25g (Dietary Fiber 2g, Sugar Alcohol 19g); Net Carbohydrates 3.6g; Protein 7g.*

Coconut Cream Pie

INGREDIENTS

1½ cups finely ground almond flour

¼ cup powdered erythritol

¼ cup butter, melted

2 cups heavy whipping cream

2 eggs plus one egg yolk

⅓ cup powdered erythritol

2 tablespoons cold butter

1 teaspoon coconut extract

¼ teaspoon liquid stevia

¼ teaspoon xanthan gum

1½ cups shredded, unsweetened coconut flakes

One 15-ounce can coconut milk, full fat, chilled

3 tablespoons powdered erythritol

DIRECTIONS

1 Make the pie crust by mixing the almond flour, ¼ cup powdered erythritol, and melted butter together until crumbly. Press the mix into the bottom of a pie pan and up the sides. Place in the fridge to firm.

2 To make the coconut filling, place the heavy whipping cream in a small saucepan and bring to a boil. Meanwhile, whisk the eggs, egg yolk, and powdered erythritol in a medium bowl. Slowly whisk the hot cream into the egg mix.

3 Transfer the egg and heavy whipping cream mix back into the small saucepan and heat over low heat, stirring constantly, for another 4 to 5 minutes or until the mix begins to thicken slightly. Remove the pan from the heat and stir in the butter, coconut extract, and liquid stevia. Sprinkle the xanthan gum over the mix and then whisk quickly to blend in well.

4 Stir in 1 cup of the coconut flakes and then pour the coconut cream into the prepared pie crust, cover, and place in the fridge to chill for at least an hour. Toast the remaining coconut until golden brown.

5 Make the topping by whisking the chilled coconut milk well until stiff peaks form. Add the powdered erythritol to the cream and whip again. Spread the coconut whipped cream over the coconut pie and then sprinkle with the toasted coconut. Slice and serve.

PER SERVING: *Calories 458; Fat 46g; Cholesterol 144mg; Sodium 52mg; Carbohydrates 22g (Dietary Fiber 2g, Sugar Alcohol 15g); Net Carbohydrates 4.6g; Protein 7g.*

NOTE: In Step 2, constantly stir the mixture so as not to cook the eggs.

Chapter **7**

Cooking Keto Cookies That Everyone Loves

Having a few good cookie recipes up your sleeve is essential as a baker, and it's just as crucial to the keto dieter. You never know when you may need to whip up a batch of cookies to bring to a party or dinner, or just to enjoy on your own. This wide range of cookie recipes in this chapter are easy to follow and give you several options. Here you can find everything from rich flavors like espresso to lighter lemon cookies that are perfect for popping in your mouth when you crave something sweet.

Lining a Cookie Tray Correctly

You may not have given much thought to how you line your cookie tray or what kind of liner you use. However, if you choose to grease a cookie tray with butter, use a piece of parchment, or reach for a silicone mat, it can make a difference in how your cookies bake. Regardless of which option you choose, you want to use something to protect your cookies from sticking to the tray. Look at the differences between a few common options, listed from most recommended to least recommended:

» **Silicone mats:** Silicone baking mats are perfect for making cookies: they're nonstick and easy to clean, and they cause the cookies to bake evenly. The silicone protects the base of the cookie from the high oven heat and also traps moisture between the cookie and the mat, making sure your cookies aren't too dry. Silicone mats and parchment can be used interchangeably, but the mats are reusable, giving them a long-term advantage.

» **Parchment paper:** Parchment paper is coated in a light silicone covering, making it safe to use in the oven. Don't worry; it won't melt. Using parchment paper on your cookie tray prevents your cookies from sticking to the tray while also acting as a barrier for direct heat. Using parchment paper prevents the bottoms of the cookies from burning, giving you a beautiful golden-brown color.

» **Butter:** Greasing a sheet tray with butter helps your cookies not stick to the tray; however, it adds extra fat to the cookies. The bottoms of the cookies get crispy because they're essentially frying in the butter as they bake, which isn't always a bad thing; it just depends on the final texture you want. Use butter when the cookies won't be in the oven too long and a crispy bottom is something you desire.

» **Foil:** Many people used to rely on foil to line a cookie sheet. Some of the advantages include making baking cookies a breeze to clean up afterward as well as being nonstick, enabling the cookies to slide right off the tray. However, foil is a heat conductor and causes the bottoms of the cookies to burn before the centers are evenly baked. We suggest you use foil only as a last resort.

🍅 Chocolate Chip Cookies

PREP TIME: 10 MIN	COOK TIME: 10 MIN	YIELD: 12 SERVINGS

INGREDIENTS

½ cup butter, softened

¾ cup granular erythritol

1 egg, room temperature

1 teaspoon vanilla extract

1½ cups finely ground almond flour

½ teaspoon baking powder

½ teaspoon sea salt

1 cup sugar-free dark chocolate chips

DIRECTIONS

1 Preheat your oven to 350 degrees F and prepare a baking tray by lining it with parchment or a silicone baking mat.

2 In a medium mixing bowl, cream the butter and the granular erythritol until well combined. Add the egg and the vanilla extract and blend again. Add the almond flour, baking powder, and sea salt and blend just until a smooth batter forms. Stir in the chocolate chips by hand.

3 Scoop the cookie dough into 12 balls and place on the prepared baking sheet.

4 Bake for 10 minutes; the cookie centers may look a little soft, but that's okay.

5 Remove from the oven and cool on a cooking rack before serving. Place in an airtight container and store at room temperature for up to one week.

PER SERVING: *Calories 152; Fat 15g; Cholesterol 38mg; Sodium 105mg; Carbohydrates 22g (Dietary Fiber 4g, Sugar Alcohol 15g); Net Carbohydrates 2.5g; Protein 3g.*

Coconut Shortbread Cookies

INGREDIENTS

⅓ cup coconut flour

⅔ cup almond flour

⅓ cup granular erythritol

¼ teaspoon baking powder

½ teaspoon xanthan gum

½ cup butter, softened

1 teaspoon vanilla extract

½ teaspoon coconut extract (optional)

DIRECTIONS

1 Prepare a baking sheet with parchment paper.

2 In a medium bowl, combine the coconut flour, almond flour, granular erythritol, baking powder, and xanthan gum. Stir to mix well. Add the softened butter, vanilla extract, and coconut extract (if using). Blend until you have a smooth, soft dough.

3 Place the dough on a piece of parchment paper, adding another piece on top. Press the dough down to flatten and then place in the fridge to chill.

4 After the dough has cooled, preheat your oven to 350 degrees F and remove the dough from the fridge and roll the dough until it's about a quarter-inch thick.

5 Cut the dough using a round 2-inch cookie cutter and place the cookies on the prepared baking sheet.

6 Bake in the preheated oven for 10 minutes or until the edges begin to turn golden brown. Remove from the oven and cool on a cooling rack. Store in an airtight container for up to two weeks.

PER SERVING: *Calories 72; Fat 7g; Cholesterol 12mg; Sodium 11mg; Carbohydrates 5g (Dietary Fiber 1g, Sugar Alcohol 3g); Net Carbohydrates .8g; Protein 1g.*

Raspberry Thumbprint Cookies

PREP TIME: 10 MIN	COOK TIME: 16 MIN	YIELD: 15 SERVINGS

INGREDIENTS

1 egg

1 teaspoon vanilla extract

½ cup butter, softened

⅔ cup granular erythritol

¼ teaspoon xanthan gum

2⅓ cups almond flour

⅛ teaspoon sea salt

½ teaspoon baking powder

⅓ cup sugar-free raspberry jam

DIRECTIONS

1 Preheat your oven to 350 degrees F and prepare a baking sheet by lining it with parchment paper. Set aside.

2 In a medium mixing bowl combine the egg, vanilla extract, butter, granular erythritol, xanthan gum, almond flour, sea salt, and baking powder. Stir well until a dough has formed.

3 Scoop the dough with a small cookie scoop or make 1½-inch balls with your hands. Place the dough on the prepared baking sheet.

4 Bake the cookies in the preheated oven for about 8 minutes.

5 Remove the cookies from the oven and press the center of each cookie with the end of a wooden spoon, making a dent. Fill the dent with a small scoop of the sugar-free raspberry jam.

6 Return the cookies to the oven and bake for another 8 minutes or until the edges begin to brown. Remove from the oven and let cool completely on the tray. The cookies will be fragile while warm so allow them to cool before enjoying. Store at room temperature for up to one week.

PER SERVING: *Calories 80; Fat 8g; Cholesterol 30mg; Sodium 35mg; Carbohydrates 10g (Dietary Fiber .6g, Sugar Alcohol 8g); Net Carbohydrates 1.2g; Protein 1g.*

🍅 Snickerdoodles

INGREDIENTS

½ cup butter, softened

½ cup granular erythritol

½ teaspoon vanilla extract

1 egg

1¼ cups almond flour

2 tablespoons coconut flour

¾ teaspoon xanthan gum

¼ teaspoon sea salt

½ teaspoon baking soda

½ teaspoon cream of tartar

2 teaspoons ground cinnamon

2 tablespoons granular erythritol

DIRECTIONS

1 Preheat your oven to 375 degrees F and prepare a baking sheet by lining it with parchment paper.

2 In a medium mixing bowl, cream the butter and ½ cup granular erythritol until light and fluffy.

3 Add the vanilla extract and the egg to the mix, scraping down the bowl to ensure all the ingredients are combined. Add the almond flour, coconut flour, xanthan gum, sea salt, baking soda, and cream of tartar and blend well to form a smooth dough. In a separate bowl, combine the cinnamon and 2 tablespoons granular erythritol and stir.

4 Scoop the cookie dough into tablespoon-sized balls and then toss them in the cinnamon mixture. After covered, place the dough on the prepared baking sheet.

5 Bake for about 6 to 8 minutes or until they're just beginning to golden. Remove from the oven and cool. Store in an airtight container for up to one week.

PER SERVING: *Calories 48; Fat 5g; Cholesterol 19mg; Sodium 40mg; Carbohydrates 6g (Dietary Fiber .5g, Sugar Alcohol 5g); Net Carbohydrates .4g; Protein 1g.*

Perfecting Cookie Storage

After you have a batch of perfect keto cookies, storing them correctly becomes important. An airtight container is always ideal, especially one that has a locking lid to seal completely. Here are a few other tips to help keep your cookies fresh after baking:

» **Allow the cookies to cool completely before locking them in an airtight container.** Excess heat can cause moisture in the air to gather inside the box or bag, soaking the cookies and making them wet and crumbly.

» **Place a piece of white bread in the container with the cookies.** The bread absorbs excess moisture and prevents the cookies from getting too soft. It also controls the humidity and helps to keep the consistency of your cookies exactly what it was when you first pulled them from the oven.

» **Keep the cookies at room temperature to prevent the texture from changing.** If you put the cookies in the fridge or freezer, the consistency will change even if you return them to room temperature before eating.

» **Store the cookies in small amounts (even individually wrapped) in zippered bags.** Only open the bag if you're ready to eat a cookie. Doing so prevents all the cookies from being exposed to air repeatedly, which can cause them to dry faster.

» **Consider baking only half of the cookie dough and storing the remaining dough already rolled into balls in the freezer.** Whenever you want fresh cookies, simply take out the cookie dough ball, thaw, and bake. You can enjoy cookies anytime you like.

Chocolate Peanut Butter Cookies

INGREDIENTS

2 tablespoons butter, melted

2 tablespoons smooth, unsweetened peanut butter

½ cup golden erythritol

1 egg

1 cup almond flour

½ teaspoon baking powder

½ teaspoon sea salt

¼ teaspoon baking soda

⅓ cup unsweetened, dark chocolate chips

DIRECTIONS

1 Preheat your oven to 350 degrees F and line a baking sheet with parchment paper.

2 Combine the butter, peanut butter, golden erythritol, and egg until smooth. Add the almond flour, baking powder, sea salt, and baking soda and mix until a batter forms. Add in the chocolate chips and stir well.

3 Scoop the dough into eight large balls and place on the prepared baking sheet.

4 Bake the cookies for 12 to 15 minutes or until the edges begin to brown slightly. Remove from the oven and cool completely on a cooking rack. Store in an airtight container for up to a week.

PER SERVING: *Calories 168; Fat 15g; Cholesterol 34mg; Sodium 201mg; Carbohydrates 20g (Dietary Fiber 4g, Sugar Alcohol 13g); Net Carbohydrates 2.8g; Protein 6g.*

Macadamia Cookies

INGREDIENTS

½ cup butter, softened

1½ cups almond flour

¼ cup granular monk fruit sweetener

¼ cup macadamia nuts, roughly chopped and toasted

2 ounces cream cheese, softened

½ teaspoon vanilla extract

DIRECTIONS

1 Preheat your oven to 325 degrees F and prepare a baking sheet with a piece of parchment paper.

2 Place the butter in a small frying pan and melt the butter over medium heat until it starts to brown (about 3 minutes). Remove from the heat and let cool to room temperature.

3 In a large bowl, mix the almond flour, granular monk fruit sweetener, macadamia nuts, cream cheese, vanilla extract, and browned butter. Stir well to form a nice batter.

4 Roll the dough into 1-inch balls and place them on the prepared baking sheet. Press down gently to flatten the cookie dough to be about a quarter-inch thick.

5 Bake for 16 minutes or until the edges start to brown. Remove from the oven, cool on a cooling rack, and then store in an airtight container for about four to five days.

PER SERVING: *Calories 116; Fat 12g; Cholesterol 26mg; Sodium 18mg; Carbohydrates 5g (Dietary Fiber 1g, Sugar Alcohol 4g); Net Carbohydrates .6g; Protein 1g.*

Lemon Sugar Cookies

PREP TIME: 10 MIN	COOK TIME: 12 MIN	YIELD: 24 COOKIES

INGREDIENTS

8 tablespoons butter, softened

¾ cup granular erythritol

2 eggs

1 tablespoon lemon juice

1 tablespoon lemon zest

1 teaspoon lemon extract

1½ cups almond flour

½ cup coconut flour

1 teaspoon baking soda

½ teaspoon xanthan gum

2 teaspoons cream of tartar

¼ teaspoon sea salt

DIRECTIONS

1 Preheat your oven to 350 degrees F and prepare a baking sheet with parchment paper.

2 In a medium mixing bowl, cream the butter, granular erythritol, eggs, lemon juice, lemon zest, and lemon extract together well. Add the almond flour, coconut flour, baking soda, xanthan gum, cream of tartar, and sea salt to the bowl and blend.

3 Scoop the cookie dough into 1-inch balls and place on the prepared sheet tray. Press the balls to flatten slightly.

4 Bake for 10 to 12 minutes or until the edges just begin to brown. Remove from the oven and move the cookies to a cooling rack. Store in an airtight container for up to one week.

PER SERVING: *Calories 93; Fat 8g; Cholesterol 28mg; Sodium 86mg; Carbohydrates 9g (Dietary Fiber 1g, Sugar Alcohol 6g); Net Carbohydrates 1.4g; Protein 2.5g.*

🍅 Cinnamon "Sugar" Cookies

PREP TIME: 30 MIN	COOK TIME: 15 MIN	YIELD: 2 DOZEN COOKIES

INGREDIENTS

½ cup butter, softened

1 cup granular erythritol

1 egg

1 teaspoon vanilla extract

2¼ cups almond flour

½ teaspoon baking soda

½ teaspoon baking powder

¼ teaspoon sea salt

2 teaspoons ground cinnamon

DIRECTIONS

1 Grease a baking sheet with butter.

2 Combine the butter, granular erythritol, egg, and vanilla extract in a medium bowl, mixing until fully blended. Add in the dry ingredients and blend until smooth. Place in the fridge to chill for about 30 minutes. Preheat the oven to 350 degrees F about 10 minutes before removing the cookie dough from the fridge.

3 Roll the batter into 1-inch balls and place on the prepared baking sheet.

4 Bake the cookies for about 12 to 15 minutes or until the edges begin to brown. Remove from the oven and cool on a cooking rack and then store in an airtight container for up to one week.

PER SERVING: *Calories 100; Fat 9g; Cholesterol 19mg; Sodium 58mg; Carbohydrates 10g (Dietary Fiber 1g, Sugar Alcohol 8g); Net Carbohydrates 1g; Protein 3g.*

☕ Double Chocolate Cookies

INGREDIENTS

1 cup smooth almond butter

⅔ cup powdered erythritol

3 tablespoons unsweetened cocoa powder

2 eggs, room temperature

1 tablespoon butter, melted

2 tablespoons water

½ tablespoon vanilla extract

1 teaspoon baking soda

⅓ cup dark, unsweetened chocolate chips

DIRECTIONS

1 Preheat your oven to 350 degrees F and prepare a baking sheet with parchment or a silicone mat.

2 Place all the ingredients, except the chocolate chips, in a large bowl and mix together using a hand mixer or stand mixer with a paddle attachment. The dough will be thick. Add the chocolate chips, folding by hand.

3 Scoop the dough into 1½ inch balls and place on the prepared baking sheet.

4 Bake the cookies for about 8 to 10 minutes and then remove from the oven. Move the cookies to a cooking rack to cool. Store in an airtight container for up to one week.

PER SERVING: *Calories 113; Fat 10g; Cholesterol 25mg; Sodium 79mg; Carbohydrates 12g (Dietary Fiber 3g, Sugar Alcohol 8g); Net Carbohydrates 1.9g; Protein 4g.*

Espresso Cookies

PREP TIME: 5 MIN | COOK TIME: 15 MIN | YIELD: 14 COOKIES

INGREDIENTS

½ cup butter, melted

¼ cup brewed espresso

¼ cup cream cheese, softened

1½ cups almond flour

¼ cup granular erythritol

1½ teaspoon ground cinnamon

1½ teaspoons finely ground espresso beans

2 teaspoons baking powder

20 drops liquid stevia

2 eggs

DIRECTIONS

1 Preheat your oven to 350 degrees F and prepare two baking sheets with parchment paper.

2 Place the melted butter and brewed espresso in a large mixing bowl and mix briefly. Mix in the softened cream cheese and blend to combine. Add the remaining ingredients, except the eggs, and blend together well. Add the eggs and blend again until the dough is uniform.

3 Scoop the dough into 14 equally sized balls and place on the prepared baking trays. Press down on the dough slightly to flatten.

4 Bake for about 12 to 15 minutes, cooking one baking tray of cookies at a time. Remove from the oven and cool the cookies completely on the baking sheet before removing. Store in an airtight container for up to one week.

PER SERVING: *Calories 142; Fat 13g; Cholesterol 48mg; Sodium 65mg; Carbohydrates 6g (Dietary Fiber 1g, Sugar Alcohol 3g); Net Carbohydrates 1.5g; Protein 4g.*

Chapter **8**

Staying Cool with Keto Ice Cream and Frozen Treats

Crafting keto ice cream and frozen treats is surprisingly easy. In fact, some of the recipes in this chapter only take a few minutes to prepare. They're simpler and less expensive than driving to the grocery and purchasing expensive keto ice cream at the store. Even better, the result is healthier without any additives or strange ingredients. Feel free to modify keto ice cream and frozen treats however you want, customizing the recipes to your personal preferences.

Going Machine-Free

Although an ice cream machine can be fun to use, many of the ice cream recipes in the following section don't require one. Instead, you mix the ingredients, pour them into an ice cube tray, and freeze them. You then blend the frozen cubes in a high-speed blender to puree the ice cubes and make for a smooth, frozen treat. No ice cream machine needed! Making ice cream has never been easier.

Chocolate Chip Ice Cream

PREP TIME: 5 HOURS PLUS 10 MIN	COOK TIME: 0 MIN	YIELD: 5 SERVINGS

INGREDIENTS

2 cups full fat coconut milk, canned

⅓ cup powdered erythritol

1 pinch sea salt

2 teaspoons vanilla extract

¼ cup finely chopped baking chocolate

2 teaspoons vodka

DIRECTIONS

1 Place the coconut milk, powdered erythritol, sea salt, and vanilla extract in a medium bowl and whisk together well. Pour the mix into an ice cube tray and place in the freezer. Freeze until solid (about 4 to 5 hours).

2 Place the ice cubes in a high-speed blender along with the vodka and blend until smooth. Place the ice cream back in the freezer to firm for at least 1 hour.

3 Divide the ice cream into bowls and top with the chopped chocolate. Gently stir in the chocolate chips and then serve immediately.

PER SERVING: Calories 78; Fat 6g; Cholesterol 0mg; Sodium 4mg; Carbohydrates 19g (Dietary Fiber 2g, Sugar Alcohol 15g); Net Carbohydrates 2.2g; Protein 1g.

Mint Chocolate Chip Ice Cream

PREP TIME: 4 HOURS PLUS 15 MIN	COOK TIME: 0 MIN	YIELD: 2 SERVINGS

INGREDIENTS

½ cup heavy whipping cream

½ medium ripe avocado

½ teaspoon vanilla extract

¾ teaspoon peppermint extract

⅛ teaspoon salt

4 tablespoons powdered erythritol

¼ cup finely chopped dark baking chocolate

1 teaspoon vodka

DIRECTIONS

1 Place all the ingredients except the chopped dark chocolate and vodka into a blender and puree until smooth.

2 Pour the mix into an ice cube tray or an airtight storage container and freeze until solid (about 3 hours depending on the size of the container you're using to freeze).

3 Place the frozen cubes into a high-speed blender and puree until smooth. Fold in the chopped chocolate by hand along with the teaspoon of vodka (this prevents the mix from freezing too hard) and then return the mixture to the freezer for another hour before serving.

PER SERVING: Calories 376; Fat 36g; Cholesterol 82mg; Sodium 151mg; Carbohydrates 44g (Dietary Fiber 9g, Sugar Alcohol 29g); Net Carbohydrates 5.9g; Protein 4g.

☕ Easy Coconut Ice Cream

PREP TIME: 5 HOURS PLUS 10 MIN

COOK TIME: 0 MIN

YIELD: 5 SERVINGS

INGREDIENTS

1 cup full fat coconut milk, canned

1 cup heavy whipping cream

⅓ cup powdered erythritol

1 pinch sea salt

2 teaspoons vanilla extract

½ cup shredded, unsweetened coconut, toasted

1 teaspoon vodka

DIRECTIONS

1 Place the coconut milk, heavy whipping cream, powdered erythritol, sea salt, and vanilla extract in a medium bowl and whisk together well. Pour the mix into an ice cube tray and place in the freezer. Freeze until solid (about 4 to 5 hours).

2 Place the ice cubes in a high-speed blender along with the vodka and blend until smooth. Return the ice cream to the freezer to firm for 1 hour.

3 Divide the ice cream into bowls and top with the unsweetened coconut. Gently stir the coconut into the mix and serve immediately.

PER SERVING: *Calories 242; Fat 25g; Cholesterol 65mg; Sodium 73mg; Carbohydrates 17g (Dietary Fiber 1g, Sugar Alcohol 13g); Net Carbohydrates 3g; Protein 2g.*

Personalizing Your Ice Cream and Frozen Treats

Nearly everyone loves ice cream, but there are so many choices that everyone prefers ice cream a bit differently. Luckily, you can alter most of the following recipes to suit your personal dessert preferences. Here are a few keto-friendly options that will keep both your taste buds and your macros equally satisfied:

- » **Berries:** A few fresh berries on top of your ice cream can add flavor without a substantial amount of carbs. These fruits are phenomenal in the summer when they're in season and perfectly ripe. A small scoop of fresh blueberries, strawberries, or raspberries can complement the Easy Coconut Ice Cream or Key Lime Pops recipe in this chapter.

- » **Unsweetened chocolate:** Mixing in a few unsweetened dark chocolate chips can take your ice cream to the next level while satisfying your chocolate cravings. Choose very finely chopped chocolate or use a peeler to shave the chocolate as thin as possible; the chocolate chunks can get pretty hard when frozen, and your dentist will thank you for making them small.

- » **Whipped cream:** Homemade keto whipped cream is fantastic on top of any ice cream. All you need is heavy whipping cream and a little powdered erythritol. Whip the cream with an electric mixer until stiff and then sprinkle in a bit of erythritol to taste. Use immediately on top of your ice cream.

- » **Sugar-free sprinkles:** A lot of sugar-free sprinkle options are available that can liven your ice cream. Grab a jar at the store and have them on hand to add a fun and exciting visual twist to your ice cream creations.

- » **Sugar-free caramel sauce:** You can make your own sugar-free caramel sauce or find it in many grocery stores near the ice cream toppings. If you make your own, opt for a recipe with erythritol, which caramelizes beautifully (many artificial sweeteners don't). Most sugar-free caramel sauces can be stored in the fridge for a few days or longer, enabling you to enjoy it on your ice cream for more than a single serving.

- » **Flavorings:** Replace vanilla extract with a different extract to make your ice cream treats even more flavorful and unique. You can use chocolate extract, coffee extract, and peppermint extract to enhance your frozen dessert.

Death By Chocolate Ice Cream

PREP TIME: 6½ HOURS | COOK TIME: 15 MIN | YIELD: 6 SERVINGS

INGREDIENTS

½ cup unsweetened cocoa powder

3 cups half-and-half

1 cup heavy whipping cream

8 egg yolks

¾ cup granular erythritol

2 teaspoons vanilla extract

½ cup finely chopped baking chocolate

DIRECTIONS

1 Place the cocoa powder, half-and-half, and heavy whipping cream in a small saucepan and whisk together. Heat over medium heat and bring to a simmer, stirring occasionally to ensure the mixture doesn't burn.

2 In a separate bowl, whisk together the egg yolks and the granular erythritol, whipping until the eggs are light and fluffy. Pour about 1 cup of the simmering cream mix into the eggs, whisking constantly. Add the egg mixture back into the saucepan and stir over low heat until the mix begins to thicken. Remove from the heat and mix in the vanilla extract.

3 Pour the ice cream mixture into an airtight container and place in the fridge to cool for at least 4 hours. After the ice cream mix has cooled, pour it into your ice cream machine and freeze the ice cream according to your machine's directions.

4 After the ice cream has reached the consistency of soft serve, fold in the chocolate, stirring gently. Place the ice cream in an airtight container and freeze for at least 2 hours before serving.

PER SERVING: *Calories 438; Fat 40g; Cholesterol 34mg; Sodium 8mg; Carbohydrates 4g (Dietary Fiber .6g, Sugar Alcohol 2.6g); Net Carbohydrates 10.8g; Protein 10.4g.*

NOTE: In Step 2, make sure you continue to whip while you pour the simmering cream mix to ensure the eggs don't cook.

🥑 Avocado Ice Cream

PREP TIME: 2 HOURS	COOK TIME: 10 MIN	YIELD: 5 SERVINGS

INGREDIENTS

1½ cups heavy whipping cream

⅓ cup powdered erythritol

½ cup chopped dark chocolate

1½ teaspoons vanilla extract

2 ripe avocados, peeled, pits removed

DIRECTIONS

1 Place the heavy whipping cream and powdered erythritol in a small saucepan and heat over medium until simmering.

2 Remove the pan from the heat and add the chocolate. Let sit for about 5 minutes and then whisk the melted chocolate into the heavy cream mix. Add the vanilla extract to the mix before pouring into a blender. Add the ripe avocado (peeled and pit removed) and puree until smooth. Refrigerate the mix until cooled completely.

3 Pour the mix into an ice cream machine and churn based on the machine's instructions. It should look similar to soft serve ice cream when ready. Transfer into an airtight container and freeze for at least two hours to firm before serving.

PER SERVING: *Calories 205; Fat 19g; Cholesterol 6mg; Sodium 7mg; Carbohydrates 31g (Dietary Fiber 10g, Sugar Alcohol 16g); Net Carbohydrates 4g; Protein 3g.*

◌ Strawberry Yogurt Pops

PREP TIME: 4 HOURS PLUS 10 MIN	COOK TIME: 0 MIN	YIELD: 8 LARGE POPS

INGREDIENTS

2 cups fresh or frozen strawberries, stems removed

1 cup full fat, canned coconut milk

1 cup plain, unsweetened Greek yogurt

¼ cup powdered erythritol

2 teaspoons vanilla extract

DIRECTIONS

1 Place all the ingredients into a blender and puree until smooth.

2 Pour the strawberry mix into a popsicle mold and place the sticks in each popsicle.

3 Freeze the popsicles until solid. Remove from the mold when you're ready to enjoy. Keep in the freezer for up to one month.

PER SERVING: *Calories 38; Fat 1g; Cholesterol 1mg; Sodium 10mg; Carbohydrates 10g (Dietary Fiber 1g, Sugar Alcohol 6g); Net Carbohydrates 3.4g; Protein 2g.*

Mocha Latte Ice Cream Bar's

PREP TIME: 4 HOURS PLUS 5 MIN	COOK TIME: 5 MIN	YIELD: 8 POPS

INGREDIENTS

1 cup heavy whipping cream

¾ cup half-and-half

¼ cup brewed espresso

⅓ cup powdered erythritol

⅓ cup unsweetened cocoa powder

1 teaspoon vanilla extract

¼ teaspoon xanthan gum

DIRECTIONS

1 Place the heavy whipping cream, half-and-half, espresso, powdered erythritol, and cocoa powder in a small saucepan and heat over medium heat. Bring to a boil and cook for 1 minute, stirring constantly. Remove from the heat and stir in the vanilla extract. Sprinkle the xanthan gum in and whisk.

2 Let the mix cool to room temperature and then pour into a popsicle mold and add the sticks to the molds.

3 Place in the freezer until frozen solid (about 3 to 4 hours). Remove from the mold when you're ready to enjoy or store in the freezer for up to one month.

PER SERVING: *Calories 143; Fat 14g; Cholesterol 49mg; Sodium 24mg; Carbohydrates 12g (Dietary Fiber 1g, Sugar Alcohol 8g); Net Carbohydrates 2.7g; Protein 2g.*

🍅 Key Lime Pops

PREP TIME: 4 HOURS PLUS 5 MIN	COOK TIME: 0 MIN	YIELD: 6 POPS

INGREDIENTS

2 ripe avocados, peeled and pit removed

½ teaspoon lime zest

¼ cup key lime juice

One 15-ounce can full fat coconut milk

½ cup powdered erythritol

10 drops liquid stevia

DIRECTIONS

1 Place all the ingredients in a blender and puree until smooth and thick. Pour into a popsicle mold and add the sticks to each pop.

2 Freeze until solid and then remove from the mold when you're ready to enjoy. Store in the freezer for about two weeks.

PER SERVING: *Calories 230; Fat 21g; Cholesterol 0mg; Sodium 17mg; Carbohydrates 25g (Dietary Fiber 5g, Sugar Alcohol 16g); Net Carbohydrates 4.4g; Protein 4g.*

Chapter 9

Baking Keto Mug, Dump, and Slow Cooker Cakes

A quick freshly baked cake can be a lifesaver, especially if you need to make a tasty treat in a hurry. You can have a cake ready to serve a crowd after just a few minutes of prep time. You can also make a cake, just for you, anytime you feel like it. This chapter has you covered with several recipes for mug cakes, dump cakes, and even slow cooker cakes. They're so easy, and all the recipes we list here keep you on track with keto.

Keeping Keto with Mug Cakes

Mug cakes are individually sized cakes that are fast and simple, enabling you to satisfy your cake craving every single night if you want. Most mug cakes are made by mixing all the ingredients inside a mug, which is then baked in the microwave for 1 to 2 minutes, allowing you to enjoy a fresh, hot cake with minimal effort.

REMEMBER

Because these cakes are cooked so quickly at such a high temperature, letting them cool for a minute or two before you take a bite is a smart idea. These little cakes are also a perfect way to make sure you control your portions and stick to your macros. Check out these easy recipes to give you your cake fix.

🍅 Vanilla Mug Cake

PREP TIME: 2 MIN	COOK TIME: 2 MIN	YIELD: 1 SERVING

INGREDIENTS

1 tablespoon coconut oil, melted

¼ cup unsweetened almond milk

½ teaspoon vanilla extract

¼ cup finely ground almond flour

1 tablespoon coconut flour

½ teaspoon baking powder

⅛ teaspoon salt

1 egg

5½ teaspoons powdered erythritol

DIRECTIONS

1 Spray a microwave-safe mug with cooking spray and then mix the melted coconut oil, almond milk, and vanilla extract in the mug. Add all the remaining ingredients to the mug and stir until nicely blended.

2 Spread the top so that it's level and then place in the microwave for 2 minutes. Let cool for 1 minute, dust with a tiny bit of powdered erythritol or one fresh berry for a garnish, and then enjoy while still warm.

PER SERVING: *Calories 402; Fat 34g; Cholesterol 212mg; Sodium 559mg; Carbohydrates 33g (Dietary Fiber 6g, Sugar Alcohol 22g); Net Carbohydrates 5.5g; Protein 14g.*

NOTE: After you mix all the ingredients in Step 1, the batter should be smooth and thick.

☕ Chocolate Chip Mug Cake

PREP TIME: 5 MIN	COOK TIME: 2 MIN	YIELD: 1 SERVING

INGREDIENTS

3 tablespoons almond flour

2 tablespoons powdered erythritol

1 tablespoon unsweetened cocoa powder

¼ teaspoon baking soda

¼ teaspoon vanilla extract

1½ tablespoons unsweetened dark chocolate chips

1 egg

1 tablespoon butter, melted

2 tablespoons heavy whipping cream

DIRECTIONS

1 Place all the dry ingredients, including the chocolate chips, into a large microwave-safe mug that you've sprayed with cooking spray. Whisk together with a fork. Add the wet ingredients and stir together until the batter is smooth.

2 Microwave for 90 seconds or until the top of the cake is firm. Let cool for a minute, top with a few extra chocolate chips, and then enjoy.

PER SERVING: *Calories 436; Fat 41g; Cholesterol 283mg; Sodium 399mg; Carbohydrates 36g (Dietary Fiber 6g, Sugar Alcohol 25g); Net Carbohydrates 5.1g; Protein 13g.*

MAKING MUG CAKES UNIQUE

After you've tried a few of the mug cake recipes in this chapter, you may be wondering how you can make them even more delicious and suited for your personal tastes. One easy way to switch things up is to change the extracts used in the recipe. For example, the Vanilla Mug Cake uses vanilla extract, but you can easily replace this with almond extract to get a tasty, almond-flavored cake. There are so many different kinds of extracts on the market, almost all of which will add no carbohydrates to the recipes.

You can also try using different flours in each mug cake recipe. A hazelnut flour, for example, would be a good substitute for an almond flour. Keep in mind that using different flours will alter the texture of the cake and change the nutritional information we have listed. However, as long as you use keto-approved flour varieties, you should be able to come up with some interesting new mug cakes that stick to your diet.

☁ Berry Lemon Mug Cake

PREP TIME: 5 MIN	COOK TIME: 2 MIN	YIELD: 1 SERVING

INGREDIENTS

1½ tablespoons butter, melted

2 tablespoons granular erythritol

¼ teaspoon vanilla extract

¼ teaspoon lemon extract

3 tablespoons heavy whipping cream

4 tablespoons almond flour

½ teaspoon baking powder

½ teaspoon lemon zest

5 blueberries

3 raspberries

DIRECTIONS

1 In a small bowl, combine the butter and granular erythritol until smooth. Stir in the vanilla extract, lemon extract, and heavy whipping cream. Add the almond flour, baking powder, and lemon zest, and mix until the batter is smooth. Gently fold in the berries and then pour the batter into a greased, large, microwave-safe bowl.

2 Microwave for 2 minutes and then let cool for 1 minute. Flip the cake out of the mug and onto a plate to show the beautiful berries and then enjoy!

PER SERVING: *Calories 486; Fat 48g; Cholesterol 107mg; Sodium 202mg; Carbohydrates 33g (Dietary Fiber 4g, Sugar Alcohol 24g); Net Carbohydrates 5.7g; Protein 8g.*

⏾ Peanut Butter Chocolate Mug Cake

PREP TIME: 5 MIN	COOK TIME: 1 MIN	YIELD: 2 SERVINGS

INGREDIENTS

2 tablespoons almond flour

1 teaspoon unsweetened cocoa powder

2 teaspoons granular erythritol

¼ teaspoon baking powder

2 eggs

1 tablespoon smooth peanut butter, unsweetened

1 tablespoon butter, melted

½ teaspoon vanilla extract

DIRECTIONS

1 In a small bowl, mix together the almond flour, unsweetened cocoa powder, granular erythritol, and baking powder. In a separate bowl, whisk together the eggs, peanut butter, melted butter, and vanilla extract until smooth. Blend the wet and dry ingredient mixes together to make a smooth batter.

2 Pour the batter into two greased microwave-safe mugs, dividing the batter evenly. Microwave the cakes, one at a time, for a minute. Let the cake cool for a minute and garnish with a few chocolate chips before enjoying.

PER SERVING: *Calories 216; Fat 18g; Cholesterol 227mg; Sodium 151mg; Carbohydrates 8g (Dietary Fiber 1.5g, Sugar Alcohol 4g); Net Carbohydrates 3g; Protein 10g.*

🥥 Coconut Mug Cake

PREP TIME: 5 MIN	COOK TIME: 2 MIN	YIELD: 1 SERVING

INGREDIENTS

2 tablespoons coconut flour

1½ teaspoons powdered erythritol

¼ teaspoon baking powder

1 pinch sea salt

1 tablespoon coconut oil, melted

1 egg

2 tablespoons canned coconut milk, full fat

1 tablespoon shredded coconut, toasted

DIRECTIONS

1 Place all the ingredients into a large, microwave-safe bowl. Whisk the mixture together well using a fork. Pour the batter into a large, greased, microwave-safe mug.

2 Bake the cake in the microwave for about 90 seconds or until the top is firm. Remove the cake from the microwave and let cool for a minute. Sprinkle with a little toasted coconut as a garnish, if desired. Enjoy while warm plain or with homemade keto whipped cream.

PER SERVING: *Calories 299; Fat 25g; Cholesterol 212mg; Sodium 443mg; Carbohydrates 20g (Dietary Fiber 6g, Sugar Alcohol 10g); Net Carbohydrates 4.5g; Protein 9g.*

NOTE: When mixing all the ingredients in Step 1, make sure the batter is smooth.

NOTE: After you remove the cake from the microwave in Step 2, the center of the cake may slightly sink.

USING YOUR OVEN TO BAKE YOUR MUG CAKE

If you love the idea of mug cakes but are hesitant to bake in the microwave, the oven is a perfectly acceptable replacement. Make sure your mug is oven-safe (most ceramic mugs are, but check the bottom of the cup to be sure) and then bake the cake in an oven that's been preheated to 350 degrees Fahrenheit for 10 to 15 minutes. The top of the cake will be firm after it's fully baked. If you double, triple, or even quadruple a mug cake recipe, dividing the batter into multiple mugs, you can bake them all at once. Making a fresh, warm, keto cake has never been easier.

Almond Butter Mug Cake

PREP TIME: 4 MIN | COOK TIME: 1 MIN | YIELD: 1 SERVING

INGREDIENTS

2½ tablespoons smooth, unsweetened almond butter

1 tablespoon granular erythritol

1 egg

¼ teaspoon vanilla extract

1 pinch sea salt

Pinch of powdered erythritol as garnish

DIRECTIONS

1 Add all the ingredients (except powdered erythritol) to a large, greased, microwave-safe mug. Stir well, using a fork, until the batter is smooth.

2 Bake in the microwave for a minute. Cool the cake for at least 30 seconds, dust with a little powdered erythritol and then enjoy.

PER SERVING: *Calories 323; Fat 27g; Cholesterol 212mg; Sodium 323mg; Carbohydrates 20g (Dietary Fiber 4g, Sugar Alcohol 12g); Net Carbohydrates 3.9g; Protein 15g.*

Whether you want to impress your guests or surprise a special someone, this Lemon Chiffon Cake in Chapter 4 is sure to steal the show.

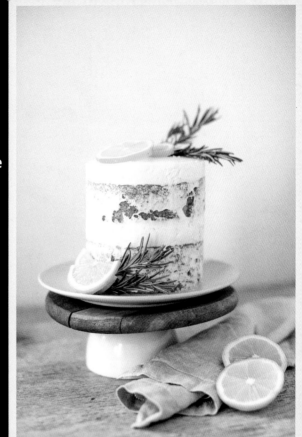

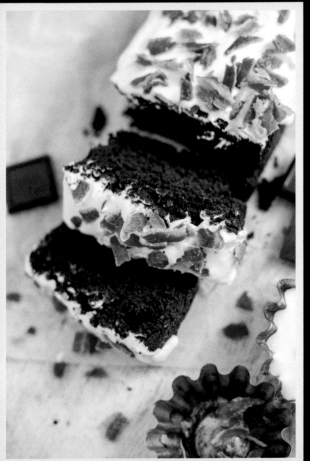

Who says bacon doesn't have a place in baking? This Chocolate Pound Cake with Bacon Bourbon Frosting in Chapter 4 is sweet and savory, all in one gorgeous package.

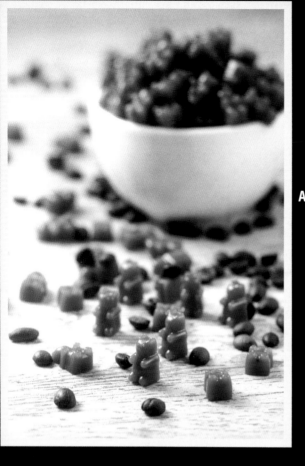

A more mature spin on a childhood classic – gummy bears with a caffeine kick! These Coffee Gummies in Chapter 5 are ultra-low-carb so you can enjoy them guilt-free.

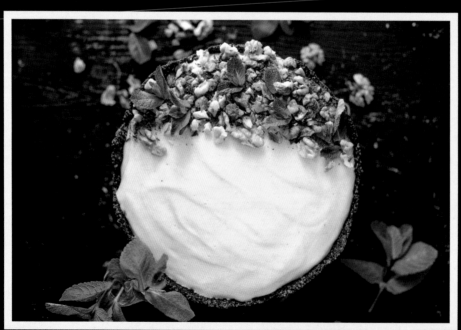

Something about the hint of mint and the aerated mousse makes this Grasshopper Mousse Pie in Chapter 6 rich yet light at the same time.

You can easily make this recipe for Raspberry Thumbprint Cookies in Chapter 7 with your little ones. After all, who doesn't love playing with their food?

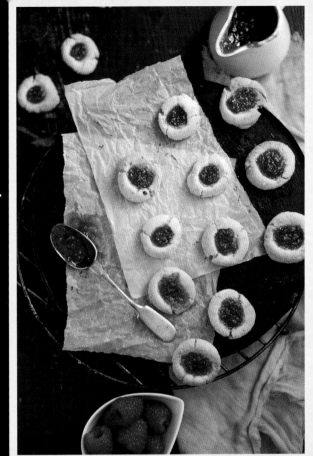

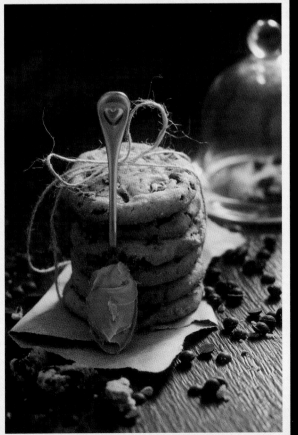

How could you go wrong with a classic recipe like chocolate chip cookies? We love adding peanut or almond butter for richness and a creamy texture as in these Chocolate Peanut Butter Cookies in Chapter 7.

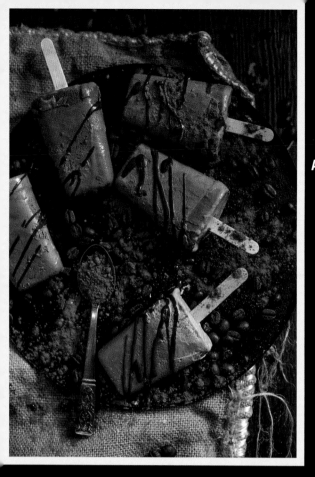

Are these Mocha Latte Ice Cream Bars in Chapter 8 dessert or breakfast? Why not both? When you have a sweet, clean treat like these, you can enjoy them day or night.

Actions speak louder than words. So show your loved ones how much you care by whipping up a batch of ultra-rich Red Velvet Doughnuts from Chapter 13.

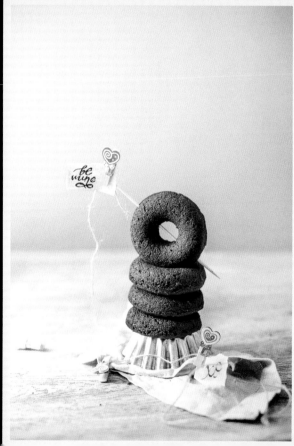

Your favorite keto dessert, spun into an easy-to-make, on-the-go friendly smoothie like this Blueberry Cheesecake Smoothie in Chapter 10. You can easily substitute your favorite berries in this recipe to make it your own.

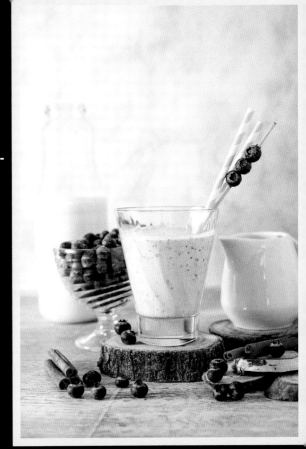

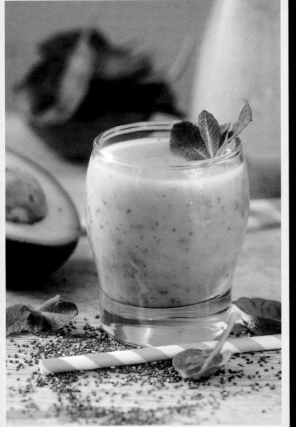

Our Green Power Smoothie in Chapter 10 is a nutrient powerhouse. And how better to get your daily dose of vitamins and minerals than in one big swig of smoothie?

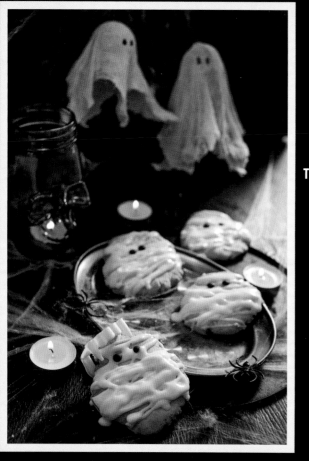

These cookies will please the kid in you. You'll have a blast making our Mummy Cookies in Chapter 14 for your next Halloween party.

Pumpkin is in season in autumn, but that doesn't mean you can't enjoy Pumpkin Crunch Cake in Chapter 15 year round. It's sweet, crunchy, and smooth all at once.

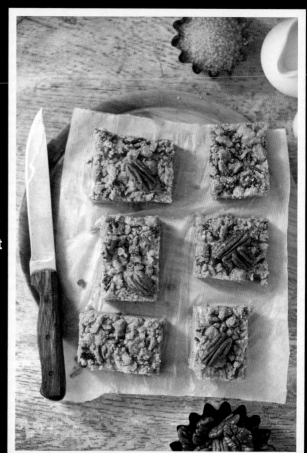

The Easter Bunny would approve of these Carrot Cake Cupcakes in Chapter 16. And so would your family when they bite into this creamy and delicate carrot cake cupcake.

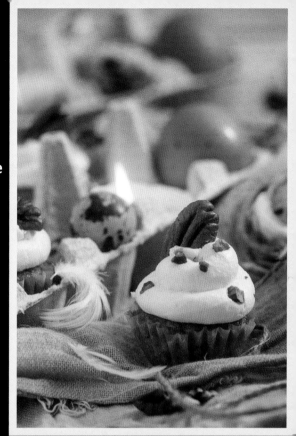

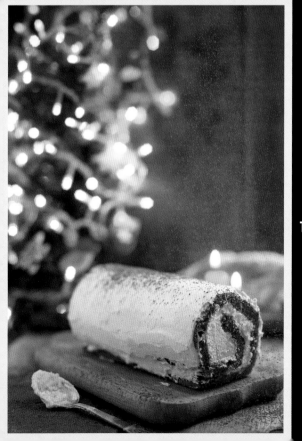

The dessert that keeps on giving. Our Gingerbread Roll Cake found in Chapter 17 is the perfect dessert recipe for the holiday season.

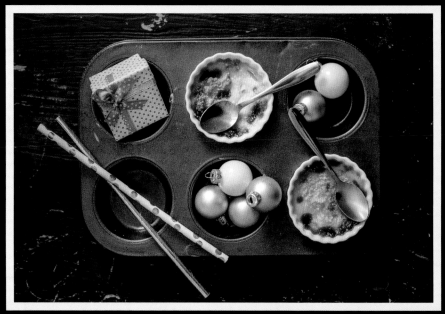

This recipe is possibly the epitome of luxury and yet so easy to make! We love the contrasting textures in our Crème Brulee recipe in Chapter 18.

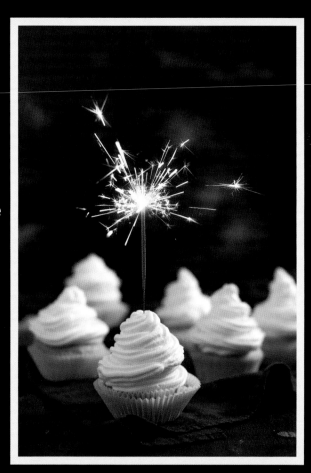

Save some of the bubbly for dessert. Add some champagne to these Champagne Cupcakes in Chapter 18 to make a super special treat for you and your family this New Year's Eve.

Tahini Chocolate Mug Cake

PREP TIME: 5 MIN	COOK TIME: 1 MIN	YIELD: 1 SERVING

INGREDIENTS

2 tablespoons finely ground almond flour

1½ tablespoons unsweetened cocoa powder

1½ teaspoons granular erythritol

¼ teaspoon baking powder

1 tablespoon tahini paste

1 egg

1 tablespoon butter, melted

2 teaspoons dark chocolate chips, unsweetened

DIRECTIONS

1 In a small bowl, combine the dry ingredients, whisking well. Add the remaining ingredients, except the dark chocolate chips, and stir until a smooth batter has formed. Fold in the chocolate chips and then scoop the batter into a large microwave-safe mug.

2 Microwave for 90 seconds or until the top of the cake is firm. Let the cake cool for a minute, sprinkle with a few extra chocolate chips and then enjoy while warm.

PER SERVING: *Calories 391; Fat 35g; Cholesterol 243mg; Sodium 181mg; Carbohydrates 22g (Dietary Fiber 8g, Sugar Alcohol 8g); Net Carbohydrates 6.3g; Protein 14.2g.*

Adding Dump and Slow Cooker Cakes to Your Keto Repertoire

Dump cakes are named quite appropriately because they involve dumping all the ingredients in a bowl, mixing them quickly, and then immediately baking the finished product. These recipes are simple and never involve creaming butter, folding ingredients, or sifting. In other words, all the difficult steps are eliminated. Dump cakes tend to be super moist and dense, which means that just a little will fill you up.

Slow cooker cakes are just as easy to put together as dump cakes, often requiring little more than mixing the ingredients until smooth. These desserts are baked inside a slow cooker with low, steady heat. To prevent the cakes from drying out, slow cooker cakes often have a flavorful liquid poured over the top, which absorbs into the cake as it bakes, keeping it moist. Choose a slow cooker cake when you want to bake a cake without the hassle of turning on the oven; simply mix the ingredients, set the timer on the slow cooker, and come back a few hours later to a perfect cake.

This section gives you a keto dump cake recipe and a couple keto slow cooker recipes.

Pumpkin Dump Cake

INGREDIENTS

¼ cup heavy whipping cream

½ cup whole milk

One 15-ounce can pumpkin puree

3 eggs

½ cup granular erythritol

2 teaspoons vanilla extract

1 tablespoon pumpkin pie spice

1 cup almond flour

⅓ cup coconut flour

½ cup granular erythritol

2 teaspoons ground cinnamon

½ cup butter, melted

DIRECTIONS

1 Preheat your oven to 350 degrees F and grease a 9x13-inch cake pan or casserole pan.

2 In a large bowl, mix the heavy whipping cream, whole milk, pumpkin puree, eggs, ½ cup granular erythritol, vanilla extract, and pumpkin pie spice. Stir until smooth. Pour the mixture into the prepared pan.

3 In a separate bowl, mix the almond flour, coconut flour, ½ cup granular erythritol, and cinnamon together. Sprinkle the mix over the pumpkin mix in the pan. Drizzle the melted butter over the entire cake pan as evenly as possible.

4 Bake in the preheated oven for about 40 minutes or until the center is firm to the touch. Let the cake cool and then slice and serve.

PER SERVING: *Calories 197; Fat 16g; Cholesterol 81mg; Sodium 36mg; Carbohydrates 24g (Dietary Fiber 3g, Sugar Alcohol 16g); Net Carbohydrates 5.1g; Protein 5g.*

🍅 Slow Cooker Lava Cake

INGREDIENTS

½ cup heavy whipping cream

4 eggs

¾ cup canned, full fat coconut milk

1 teaspoon vanilla extract

¼ cup butter, melted

1 cup finely ground almond flour

¼ cup unsweetened cocoa powder

4 tablespoons granular erythritol

2 teaspoons baking powder

¼ teaspoon sea salt

½ cup unsweetened dark chocolate chips

½ cup water

2 tablespoons unsweetened cocoa powder

1 tablespoon granular erythritol

DIRECTIONS

1 Grease the ceramic insert of your slow cooker.

2 In a large bowl, combine the heavy whipping cream, eggs, coconut milk, vanilla extract, and melted butter. Add the almond flour, cocoa powder, 4 tablespoons granular erythritol, baking powder, and salt and stir until a thick batter forms. Pour the batter into the slow cooker bowl and spread to smooth. Sprinkle the dark chocolate chips over the top of the batter.

3 In a small bowl, combine the water, 2 tablespoons cocoa powder, and 1 tablespoon granular erythritol. Heat the mix for about 30 seconds in the microwave to dissolve the sweetener.

4 Pour the water mix over the top of the cake batter and then cover the slow cooker and bake on the low setting for 2 hours. Let cool slightly before slicing and serving

PER SERVING: *Calories 372; Fat 34g; Cholesterol 189mg; Sodium 262mg; Carbohydrates 27g (Dietary Fiber 8g, Sugar Alcohol 13g); Net Carbohydrates 6.3g; Protein 11g.*

NOTE: The cake is done and ready to enjoy when the top is shiny and fudgelike.

☕ Lemon Coconut Slow Cooker Cake

PREP TIME: 10 MIN	COOK TIME: 3 HOURS	YIELD: 8 SERVINGS

INGREDIENTS

1½ cups almond flour

½ cup coconut flour

3 tablespoons granular erythritol

2 teaspoons baking powder

½ teaspoon xanthan gum

½ cup coconut oil, melted

½ cup heavy whipping cream

2 tablespoons lemon juice

2 teaspoons lemon zest

2 eggs

3 tablespoons granular erythritol

½ cup hot water

2 tablespoons butter

2 tablespoons lemon juice

DIRECTIONS

1 In a medium bowl, whisk together the almond flour, coconut flour, 3 tablespoons granular erythritol, baking powder, and xanthan gum. Add the melted coconut oil, heavy whipping cream, 2 tablespoons lemon juice, lemon zest, and eggs to the dry ingredients and mix well to form a smooth batter. Spread the batter into your slow cooker insert.

2 In a small bowl, combine the remaining 3 tablespoons granular erythritol, hot water, butter, and 2 tablespoons lemon juice. Stir to melt the butter and then pour the mix over the cake batter in the slow cooker.

3 Cover the slow cooker and bake on the high setting for 2 to 3 hours or until a toothpick comes out of the center of the cake cleanly. Serve warm.

PER SERVING: *Calories 369; Fat 35g; Cholesterol 81mg; Sodium 133mg; Carbohydrates 19g (Dietary Fiber 5g, Sugar Alcohol 9g); Net Carbohydrates 4.6g; Protein 8g.*

Chapter **10**

Blending Keto Shakes and Smoothies

S hakes and smoothies can serve so many purposes. They're great for breakfast, a perfect midday snack, and a fantastic, sweet treat at the end of the day. Just because you're doing keto doesn't mean that you have to go without. There are lots of delicious keto-approved shakes and smoothies, and you'll never grow tired of them. In fact, with these recipes on hand, you can look forward to your cool thick drink all day long.

Many of our recipes contain almond milk or other nut milks. If you happen to have a nut allergy, feel free to substitute unsweetened coconut milk or any of your favorite keto milks. The recipes will still taste just as delicious!

In addition, be sure to use the correct coconut milk as specified in each recipe. Canned coconut milk is much more rich, heavy, and higher in fat than the refrigerated cartons of coconut milk. Some recipes benefit from the thickness of canned coconut milk and that is why we use it! They truly are very different ingredients so be sure to grab the right one!

We suggest you avoid cream of coconut, which is more of a concentrated drink mix meant more for mixing drinks than making keto shakes and smoothies. Cream of coconut typically contains tons of sugar, so make sure to skip it and find real coconut cream.

Shaking Up Your Keto Diet with Shakes

Everyone loves a good shake and luckily, there are plenty that you can enjoy on a keto diet. Although you may think of a shake as containing ice cream and, therefore, being full of sugar, that doesn't have to be the case. Shakes can be made with all kinds of ingredients in order to give you a thick, creamy, cold dessert that will fill you up and cool you down. These recipes are also perfect for enjoying on the go so grab your to-go cup, a straw, and your blender and start enjoying these delicious, easy-to-make desserts.

Peanut Butter Chocolate Milkshake

PREP TIME: 2 HOURS AND 5 MIN	COOK TIME: 2 MINS	YIELD: 3 SERVINGS

INGREDIENTS

1 cup heavy whipping cream

1½ cups unsweetened almond milk

6 tablespoons powdered erythritol

¼ cup smooth peanut butter, unsweetened

3 tablespoons unsweetened cocoa powder

1 teaspoon vanilla extract

DIRECTIONS

1 Add all the ingredients to a small saucepan and heat to a simmer, whisking together until smooth. Remove from the heat and cool slightly.

2 Pour the mix into an ice cube tray and freeze until hardened.

3 Place the ice cubes in a blender and puree until smooth and thick. Add a splash of almond milk if needed to help blend. Pour into glasses and serve.

PER SERVING: *Calories 425; Fat 42g; Cholesterol 109mg; Sodium 64mg; Carbohydrates 35g (Dietary Fiber 3g, Sugar Alcohol 24g); Net Carbohydrates 7.5g; Protein 8g.*

⌖ Almond Butter Shake

INGREDIENTS

1½ cups unsweetened almond milk

2 tablespoons smooth almond butter, unsweetened

1 cup ice cubes

1 tablespoon unsweetened cocoa powder

1 tablespoon chia seeds

8 drops liquid stevia

½ ripe avocado, peeled and pit removed

DIRECTIONS

1   Add all the ingredients to blender and puree until smooth.

2   Pour the shake into two cups and enjoy immediately.

PER SERVING: *Calories 242; Fat 20g; Cholesterol 0mg; Sodium 133mg; Carbohydrates 13g (Dietary Fiber 9g, Sugar Alcohol 0g); Net Carbohydrates 4.4g; Protein 7g.*

Strawberry Shake

INGREDIENTS

¼ cup full fat, canned coconut milk

¾ cup almond milk, unsweetened

½ cup frozen chopped strawberries

1 tablespoon coconut oil

½ teaspoon vanilla extract

DIRECTIONS

1 Add all the ingredients to a blender and puree until smooth.

2 Pour into a glass and enjoy immediately.

PER SERVING: *Calories 301; Fat 29g; Cholesterol 0mg; Sodium 137mg; Carbohydrates 11g (Dietary Fiber 3g, Sugar Alcohol 0g); Net Carbohydrates 8g; Protein 3g.*

⊙ Coconut Vanilla Shake

PREP TIME: 5 MIN	COOK TIME: 0 MINS	YIELD: 4 SERVINGS

INGREDIENTS

2 cups unsweetened, refrigerated coconut milk

1 cup heavy whipping cream

6 tablespoons powdered erythritol

1 teaspoon coconut extract (optional)

2 teaspoons vanilla extract or vanilla bean paste

2 cups ice cubes

2 tablespoons unsweetened shredded coconut, toasted

DIRECTIONS

1 Add all the ingredients, except the shredded coconut, to a blender and puree until smooth.

2 Pour into four glasses and garnish with the shredded, toasted coconut and enjoy.

PER SERVING: *Calories 254; Fat 26g; Cholesterol 82mg; Sodium 29mg; Carbohydrates 21g (Dietary Fiber .5g, Sugar Alcohol 18g); Net Carbohydrates 2.7g; Protein 2g.*

Living Your Keto Life with Smoothies

Many keto dieters love the convenience and delicious taste of smoothies. You can add almost anything to a smoothie, which makes it a versatile option. Because blending the ingredients is usually all you need to do in order to make a great smoothie, you can whip up and quickly enjoy these recipes. Easy keto desserts are often the best.

Smoothies differ from shakes because they tend to be less rich and have more nutrient-rich ingredients. For example, you may commonly see flaxseeds or hempseeds in a smoothie whereas these ingredients aren't often present in a shake. Smoothies are also a little less rich than a shake and therefore aren't only perfect for a nice light dessert, but they're also great as a breakfast, lunch, or snack option.

MAKING SHAKES AND SMOOTHIES THICK

Although making a smoothie requires little in the way of actual cooking, it can be tricky to achieve the perfect texture. A shake should be thick with a smooth, creamy texture, while still being fluid enough to drink through a straw easily. It should be icy cold, but not frozen solid. We created these recipes so that you'll get perfect shake and smoothie results every time, and here are a few tips to help you achieve that ideal texture:

- **Frozen fruit:** If your smoothie or milkshake recipe calls for fruit (berries are used most frequently in low-carb recipes), be sure to freeze it beforehand. Frozen fruit helps chill the smoothie or shake and preserves a lot of flavor because you don't need to water it down by adding ice. Keep frozen fruit ready in your freezer so you never have to wait for that treat.

- **Avocado:** Avocado is a perfect smoothie and milkshake ingredient for a variety of reasons. First, avocados are wonderfully healthy, adding beneficial fats, vitamins, and minerals to your drink. To get a smooth, uniform consistency in a smoothie, you need a thickening agent. Many smoothie shops use bananas for this, but avocadoes are even better (as well as being low-carb). The fats from the avocado help create the exact consistency you want in your smoothie or shake.

- **Frozen liquids:** Anytime your smoothie or milkshake recipe calls for milk, coffee, or any other liquid, plan ahead and make ice cubes using this ingredient. Pop them out and use the frozen cubes in the smoothie to help chill the drink, thicken it, and avoid altering the flavor by watering it down. Using frozen cubes does take a little bit of planning, but it's definitely worth it.

Green Power Smoothie

INGREDIENTS

1 tablespoon chia seeds

½ cup canned coconut milk

½ cup plain Greek yogurt

1½ cups unsweetened almond milk

¼ cup vanilla whey protein powder

1 ripe avocado, peeled and pit removed

1 cup baby spinach

1 cup chopped kale

¼ cup fresh mint leaves

1 cup ice cubes

½ teaspoon vanilla extract

DIRECTIONS

1 Add all the ingredients to a blender and puree until smooth.

2 Pour into two glasses and serve immediately.

PER SERVING: *Calories 464; Fat 35g; Cholesterol 20mg; Sodium 245mg; Carbohydrate 22g (Dietary Fiber 12g, Sugar Alcohol 0g); Net Carbohydrate 10g; Protein 21g.*

ADDING SUPERFOODS TO YOUR SMOOTHIE

You can easily add superfoods (such as blueberries) to your smoothies, sticking to your keto diet while getting a few extra nutrients into your system. We love adding ingredients that blend right into smoothies without altering the flavor, which means you can add them anytime!

If you're looking to increase the protein content of your smoothie, try adding some hulled hemp seeds. You can obtain a little extra fiber by blending a tablespoon of ground flaxseeds into your smoothie. Chia seeds are loaded with antioxidants as well as plant-based proteins. Try any of these (or all of them) in any of these recipes to give the smoothies a power boost!.

🍅 Cinnamon Vanilla Smoothie

PREP TIME: 5 MIN	COOK TIME: 0 MINS	YIELD: 1 SERVING

INGREDIENTS

½ cup canned coconut milk

½ cup almond milk

1 cup ice

1 tablespoon coconut oil

½ teaspoon ground cinnamon

¼ cup vanilla whey protein powder, sugar-free and low-carb

1 teaspoon vanilla extract

DIRECTIONS

1 Add all the ingredients to a blender and puree until smooth.

2 Pour into a glass and enjoy.

PER SERVING: *Calories 246; Fat 16g; Cholesterol 20mg; Sodium 176mg; Carbohydrates 5g (Dietary Fiber 3g, Sugar Alcohol 0g); Net Carbohydrates 2.6g; Protein 19g.*

PLANNING AHEAD FOR SMOOTHIES AND SHAKES

A great thing about keto smoothies and shakes is that you can prepare almost all the ingredients ahead of time and can even pre-make the smoothies and shakes. Pick a recipe that you love and double or triple it. Enjoy one right then and pour the excess into an ice cube tray or small silicone mold (fat bomb molds work wonderfully). Cover the tray and place it in the freezer. The next time you want a shake or smoothie, just put the cubes in the blender and puree until smooth. You may need to use a small splash of unsweetened milk or water to get the cubes blending well. Also, the smoothies that contain avocado or other green veggies may turn slightly brown when frozen. Don't worry; that's just oxidation, and they'll still taste great.

⊙ Strawberry Avocado Smoothie

PREP TIME: 2 MIN	COOK TIME: 0 MINS	YIELD: 5 SERVINGS

INGREDIENTS

1 pound strawberries, frozen

1 cup unsweetened almond milk

½ cup heavy whipping cream

1 ripe avocado, peeled and pit removed

¼ cup granular erythritol

DIRECTIONS

1 Place all the ingredients in a blender and puree until smooth.

2 Pour into glasses and serve while cold.

PER SERVING: *Calories 183; Fat 16g; Cholesterol 33mg; Sodium 47mg; Carbohydrates 21g (Dietary Fiber 5g, Sugar Alcohol 9g); Net Carbohydrates 6.8g; Protein 2g.*

Mocha Smoothie

INGREDIENTS

½ cup coconut milk

1½ cups unsweetened almond milk

1 teaspoon vanilla extract

3 tablespoons granular erythritol and monk fruit blend

¼ cup brewed espresso

3 tablespoons unsweetened cocoa powder

1 ripe avocado, peeled and pit removed

DIRECTIONS

1 Pour the espresso into an ice cube tray and freeze until solid.

2 Place all the ingredients, including the espresso ice cubes, into a blender and puree until smooth.

3 Pour into glasses and serve while cold.

PER SERVING: *Calories 151; Fat 13g; Cholesterol 0mg; Sodium 96mg; Carbohydrates 23g (Dietary Fiber 7g, Sugar Alcohol 12g); Net Carbohydrates 3.6g; Protein 3g.*

Blueberry Cheesecake Smoothie

| PREP TIME: 5 MIN | COOK TIME: 0 MINS | YIELD: 1 SERVING |

INGREDIENTS

1 cup unsweetened almond milk

2 ounces cream cheese

⅛ cup heavy whipping cream

½ teaspoon ground cinnamon

1 teaspoon vanilla extract

½ cup frozen blueberries

1 tablespoon granular erythritol

DIRECTIONS

1 Place the almond milk, cream cheese, and heavy whipping cream in a blender and puree until the cream cheese is fully mixed into the milk.

2 Place the remaining ingredients into the blender and puree until smooth.

3 Pour into glasses, garnish with a few more blueberries and serve chilled.

PER SERVING: *Calories 391; Fat 33g; Cholesterol 103mg; Sodium 390mg; Carbohydrates 30g (Dietary Fiber 4g, Sugar Alcohol 12g); Net Carbohydrates 14g; Protein 6g.*

Pineapple Kale Smoothie

INGREDIENTS

2 cups chopped baby kale

¾ cup unsweetened almond milk

½ ripe avocado, peeled and pit removed

¼ cup plain, unsweetened Greek yogurt

¼ cup frozen pineapple chunks

2 teaspoons granular erythritol

DIRECTIONS

1 Place all the ingredients into a blender and puree until smooth.

2 Pour into two glasses and serve while cold.

PER SERVING: *Calories 168; Fat 11g; Cholesterol 5mg; Sodium 110mg; Carbohydrates 19g (Dietary Fiber 7g, Sugar Alcohol 4g); Net Carbohydrates 8.5g; Protein 7g.*

Chapter **11**

Keeping Warm with Keto Hot Drinks

Nothing's better than starting your day with a perfect cup of coffee, and these recipes not only do that, but they also give you some tasty coffee and cocoa options that are completely dessert-worthy. Our keto recipes not only help you get your morning coffee fix, but they also give you a boost of healthy fats paired with incredible flavors. All the beverages in this chapter are best when served warm. They're rich, satisfying, and still keto-friendly — everything you need to warm your soul on a cold, wintery day.

Making Some Classic Keto Coffee Drinks

There are a lot of great, flavored coffee drinks out there that you may miss when you start following a keto diet. A traditional vanilla-flavored coffee from your local coffee shop may surprisingly contain a lot of carbs. Fortunately, there are plenty of ways to make your coffee favorites keto-friendly. We use various methods to infuse coffees with flavor and also utilize alternative sugars to give them that sweet taste you want. The classic keto coffee drinks can still be yours, and we have the recipes in this section to make that happen.

Turmeric Vanilla Power Coffee

PREP TIME: 2 MIN	COOK TIME: 0 MIN	YIELD: 1 SERVING

INGREDIENTS

8 ounces hot brewed coffee

½ cup unsweetened almond milk

1 teaspoon coconut oil

½ teaspoon ground turmeric

1 teaspoon vanilla extract

1 teaspoon butter

DIRECTIONS

1 Place all the ingredients in a blender and puree for about 10 seconds to emulsify the oils and butter into the coffee. Pour into a mug and enjoy while hot.

PER SERVING: *Calories 110; Fat 10g; Cholesterol 10mg; Sodium 91mg; Carbohydrates 3g (Dietary Fiber 1g, Sugar Alcohol 0g); Net Carbohydrates 1.9g; Protein 1g.*

🍅 Vanilla Keto Coffee

PREP TIME: 5 MIN | COOK TIME: 0 MIN | YIELD: 1 SERVING

INGREDIENTS

8 ounces brewed coffee

½ teaspoon vanilla extract

1 teaspoon coconut oil

⅛ teaspoon ground cinnamon

DIRECTIONS

1 Place all the ingredients in a blender and puree for 10 seconds to combine everything well.

2 Pour into a mug and serve while hot.

PER SERVING: *Calories 54; Fat 5g; Cholesterol 0mg; Sodium 5mg; Carbohydrates 1g (Dietary Fiber 0g, Sugar Alcohol 0g); Net Carbohydrates .6g; Protein 0g.*

NOTE: For extra flavor, use vanilla bean paste instead of vanilla extract.

Hazelnut Keto Coffee

PREP TIME: 10 MIN	COOK TIME: 5 MIN	YIELD: 2 SERVINGS

INGREDIENTS

2 cups brewed coffee

½ cup whole hazelnuts, toasted

2 tablespoons butter

½ teaspoon ground cinnamon

DIRECTIONS

1   Place the brewed coffee and hazelnuts in a small saucepan. Bring to a boil and then remove from the heat, cover, and let sit for 30 minutes. Strain the coffee, removing and discarding the hazelnuts.

2   Bring the coffee to a boil again and then pour into a blender along with the butter and cinnamon. Blend for 5 seconds to combine and then pour into a mug and enjoy.

PER SERVING: *Calories 105; Fat 12g; Cholesterol 30mg; Sodium 5mg; Carbohydrates .5g (Dietary Fiber 0g, Sugar Alcohol 0g); Net Carbohydrates .2g; Protein .3g.*

TIP: If you're wary of discarding the hazelnuts, wrap them well and store them in the fridge for up to one week. Add the nuts to a smoothie or puree them to make hazelnut butter.

VARY IT: You can also replace the hazelnuts in this recipe completely, using 1 tablespoon of sugar-free Torani hazelnut syrup in its place.

☕ Cinnamon Keto Latte

INGREDIENTS

¾ cup unsweetened almond milk

1 tablespoon cream cheese, softened

2 tablespoons granular erythritol

2 teaspoons ground cinnamon

1 teaspoon vanilla extract

¼ cup brewed espresso

DIRECTIONS

1 Place the almond milk, cream cheese, granular erythritol, and cinnamon in a small pot. Heat over medium heat, stirring frequently, and let the cream cheese melt and mix into the milk.

2 Remove from the heat after the mix is uniform and then stir in the vanilla extract and brewed espresso. Pour into a mug and enjoy while hot.

PER SERVING: *Calories 107; Fat 7g; Cholesterol 16mg; Sodium 190mg; Carbohydrates 32g (Dietary Fiber 4g, Sugar Alcohol 24g); Net Carbohydrates 4.5g; Protein 2g.*

Mocha Mint Latte

INGREDIENTS

1½ cups unsweetened, canned coconut milk

½ cup fresh mint leaves

2½ tablespoons cocoa powder, unsweetened

1 tablespoon granular erythritol

¼ cup brewed espresso

1 sugar-free peppermint stick (optional)

DIRECTIONS

1 Place the coconut milk and mint leaves in a small saucepan and bring to a boil. Remove from the heat, cover, and let sit for 30 minutes.

2 Strain and discard the mint leaves and place the infused coconut milk back into the saucepan along with the cocoa powder and granular erythritol. Bring to a simmer over medium heat. Add the espresso to the pot, stir, and then pour the latte into a mug.

3 Garnish with the peppermint stick if desired and enjoy while hot.

PER SERVING: *Calories 112; Fat 9g; Cholesterol 0mg; Sodium 31mg; Carbohydrates 24g (Dietary Fiber 6g, Sugar Alcohol 12g); Net Carbohydrates 5.6g; Protein 4g.*

🍅 Golden Milk Cappuccino

PREP TIME: 5 MIN	COOK TIME: 10 MIN	YIELD: 4 SERVINGS

INGREDIENTS

2 cups coconut milk, full fat, canned

2 cups unsweetened almond milk

2 tablespoons ground turmeric

1 teaspoon ground cinnamon

1 teaspoon ground ginger

1 teaspoon vanilla extract

2 tablespoons granular erythritol

2 tablespoons coconut oil

½ cup brewed espresso

DIRECTIONS

1 Add the milks, turmeric, cinnamon, ginger, vanilla extract, and granular erythritol in a small saucepan and bring to a boil. Boil for 5 minutes and then remove from the heat and let the mixture sit for 5 minutes.

2 Add the coconut oil to the pan and pour into a blender. Blend the mix for 10 seconds.

3 Divide the hot, brewed espresso between four mugs and pour the hot milk mixture over the espresso. Enjoy while hot.

PER SERVING: *Calories 323; Fat 33g; Cholesterol 0mg; Sodium 106mg; Carbohydrates 15g (Dietary Fiber 2g, Sugar Alcohol 6g); Net Carbohydrates 7g; Protein 4g.*

Hot Buttered Rum

PREP TIME: 2 MIN	COOK TIME: 3 MIN	YIELD: 6 SERVINGS

INGREDIENTS

⅔ cup butter

1 anise star

1 tablespoon ground cinnamon

½ teaspoon ground ginger

½ teaspoon ground nutmeg

½ teaspoon ground allspice

1 teaspoon vanilla extract

¼ cup golden erythritol

¾ cup water

¼ cup heavy whipping cream

½ cup rum

DIRECTIONS

1 In a large pot, melt the butter along with the anise star over medium heat. Add the remaining spices to the pot with the butter mixture and stir well. Add the water and heavy whipping cream to the pot and stir.

2 Let the mixture simmer for 5 minutes and then remove from the heat.

3 Add the rum and stir well. Serve hot.

PER SERVING: *Calories 264; Fat 25g; Cholesterol 67mg; Sodium 4mg; Carbohydrates 10g (Dietary Fiber 1g, Sugar Alcohol 8g); Net Carbohydrates 1g; Protein 0g.*

Adding Cocoa Recipes to Your Keto Repertoire

A rich, warm cup of cocoa is something that everyone longs for once in a while, which is why we crafted some delicious cocoa recipes that will fit right into your keto diet plan. Our recipes in this section use unsweetened cocoa powder or unsweetened dark chocolate chips as the primary chocolate flavor, none of which will add any carbohydrates to the drink. Of course, as with any cup of hot cocoa, you can take each of these recipes to the next level when topped with a keto whipped cream.

Although our first cocoa recipe sticks to the basic, delicious chocolate taste that you automatically think of when you hear the word "cocoa," the other recipes add a little flair. With a little spice in one and a little tropical taste in the other, there is a perfect keto cocoa recipe here for everyone.

⬤ Keto Hot Cocoa

PREP TIME: 2 MIN	COOK TIME: 3 MIN	YIELD: 1 SERVING

INGREDIENTS

1 cup unsweetened almond milk

2 tablespoons heavy whipping cream

2 tablespoons powdered erythritol

1 tablespoon unsweetened cocoa powder

¼ teaspoon vanilla extract

1 pinch sea salt

DIRECTIONS

1 Place the almond milk, heavy whipping cream, powdered erythritol, and cocoa powder in a small saucepan and heat over medium heat, whisking frequently until simmering.

2 Remove from the heat and stir in the vanilla extract and sea salt. Pour into a glass and enjoy while hot.

PER SERVING: *Calories 155; Fat 14g; Cholesterol 41mg; Sodium 543mg; Carbohydrates 31g (Dietary Fiber 3g, Sugar Alcohol 24g); Net Carbohydrates 3.5g; Protein 3g.*

INFUSING MILK WITH FLAVOR

This chapter has many recipes that require infusing milk to add flavor to your hot drink. Doing so is a great way to get the taste you want without any added carbs or calories. Almost any milk can be infused, making it the perfect foundation for a variety of hot keto drinks. Start with the mixes we recommend, but don't be afraid to experiment with your own blends of nuts and spices. Here are a few ideas to help you create a hot milk infusion:

- **Nuts:** Infusing milk with nuts makes for a deep, rich flavor without any additional carbs. Use ¼ cup of nuts with 1 cup of keto-friendly milk. You should always toast the nuts first for optimal flavor and then bring the liquid to a boil and add the nuts. Remove the mixture from the heat and then cover it and let it sit for at least 30 minutes. You can make this longer if you would like a richer flavor. Strain and discard the nuts or puree them into a nut butter to use later.

- **Whole spices:** Cinnamon sticks, star anise, whole cloves, and whole nutmeg are popular options that can add a tremendous amount of flavor. Using whole spices rather than ground spices prevents your beverage from having spice particles while still retaining the overall character. Whole spices tend to create a fresher flavor, whereas ground spices tend to lose their flavor over time because they're exposed to more air.

- **Fresh herbs:** Although the idea of chewing a mint leaf while drinking your coffee may sound a bit odd, don't be afraid to try something new and see what you think. Boil the milk of your choice with a few mint leaves, basil leaves, or even fresh rosemary. After straining, you'll have a delicious flavored milk that adds a wonderful, subtle taste to your hot beverage.

Mexican Hot Chocolate

| PREP TIME: 5 MIN | COOK TIME: 5 MIN | YIELD: 3 SERVINGS |

INGREDIENTS

One 15-ounce canned coconut milk, full fat

½ cup dark, unsweetened chocolate chips

4 tablespoons granular erythritol

½ teaspoon vanilla extract

¼ cup heavy whipping cream

½ cup water

1 teaspoon ground cinnamon

¼ teaspoon ground chili powder

⅛ teaspoon ground cloves

DIRECTIONS

1 Place all the ingredients into a small saucepan and heat over medium heat. Whisk constantly to ensure the chocolate doesn't burn and blends evenly into the mix.

2 After the mixture begins to steam and the chocolate is completely incorporated, pour into mugs and enjoy while hot.

PER SERVING: *Calories 452; Fat 47g; Cholesterol 27mg; Sodium 33mg; Carbohydrates 40g (Dietary Fiber 9g, Sugar Alcohol 22g); Net Carbohydrates 8.9g; Protein 5g.*

🥥 Coconut Cocoa

INGREDIENTS

2 cups canned coconut milk, full fat

4 tablespoons heavy whipping cream

¼ cup shredded, unsweetened coconut

4 tablespoons powdered erythritol

2 tablespoons unsweetened cocoa powder

½ teaspoon vanilla extract

1 pinch sea salt

¼ teaspoon coconut extract (optional)

DIRECTIONS

1 Place the coconut milk and heavy whipping cream in a small saucepan along with the shredded coconut. Bring to a boil and then remove from the heat. Cover the pan and let sit for 30 minutes to infuse the milks with more coconut flavor.

2 Strain the coconut from the milk, discarding the shredded coconut and returning the milk to the pan. Add the powdered erythritol and cocoa powder to the pan and whisk well.

3 Heat over medium heat until the mix just begins to simmer, whisking constantly. Turn off the heat and add the vanilla extract, sea salt, and coconut extract (if using). Whisk well. Pour into glasses and enjoy while hot.

PER SERVING: *Calories 422; Fat 45g; Cholesterol 27mg; Sodium 114mg; Carbohydrates 25g (Dietary Fiber 2g, Sugar Alcohol 16g); Net Carbohydrates 6.6g; Protein 5g.*

EMPHASIZING CONVENIENCE

Although all the drinks in this chapter are best when enjoyed hot, you can take a few steps to make them a keto drink later on. For example, you can infuse milk ahead of time and keep it in the fridge until you're ready to use it. You can also cold brew coffee in advance and heat it when you want a festive cup of java. You can double or triple all the cocoa recipes in this chapter to make large batches. Store the cocoa in the fridge and reheat it anytime you would like a warm mug of delicious keto chocolate.

Chapter **12**

Serving Up Keto Cocktails

Many cocktails and alcoholic beverages are full of hidden sugars. Even the average can of beer has 13 grams of carbs. When you're on the keto diet, knowing what drinks you can responsibly enjoy and which you should avoid isn't easy. Never fear, our dear reader. This chapter has you covered with some keto cocktails, many of which can be great dessert cocktails. Here you can find some phenomenal keto drink recipes that you're sure to love. There's something for everyone, no matter their drink preference.

Making Favorite Cocktails the Keto Way

A delicious cocktail is a perfect way to end a meal or end the day, and fortunately for you, a lot of fantastic cocktail options fit right into a balanced keto diet. You don't need all the carbs that traditional cocktails contain to have a classy or fun drink!

The following recipes are classic cocktails that are keto-approved. They stick with low-carb (or no-carb) alcohols and use fruits and herbs that are low-carb. When needed, we add some liquid stevia or erythritol to give the cocktail a little sweetness, making it super easy to drink. You're going to love the cocktail classics and our few cocktail creations in the following section.

Vanilla Vodka Mojito

PREP TIME: 2 MIN	COOK TIME: 0 MIN	YIELD: 1 SERVING

INGREDIENTS

4 mint leaves, fresh

2 tablespoons lime juice

¼ teaspoon granular erythritol

1½ ounces vodka

¼ teaspoon vanilla extract

¼ cup club soda

½ cup ice cubes

DIRECTIONS

1 Place the mint leaves, lime juice, and granular erythritol in a cocktail shaker and muddle to crush the mint leaves with the erythritol and lime juice.

2 Add ice first followed by vodka and vanilla extract to the glass, cover, and shake for about 30 seconds.

3 Pour the vodka mix into a tall glass with the ice cubes from the shaker.

4 Top with the club soda and garnish with an extra mint leaf and lime slice. Serve and enjoy.

PER SERVING: *Calories 41; Fat 0g; Cholesterol 0mg; Sodium 13mg; Carbohydrates 3g (Dietary Fiber 0g, Sugar Alcohol 1g); Net Carbohydrates 2g; Protein 0g.*

VARY IT: If you don't have clear vanilla, regular vanilla extract works fine, although it gives the drink a slight brown tint. You can also use fresh vanilla bean seeds scraped from one vanilla bean.

🍊 Orange Margarita

PREP TIME: 2 MIN	COOK TIME: 0 MIN	YIELD: 2 SERVINGS

INGREDIENTS

¾ cup tequila

¼ cup lime juice

1½ teaspoons orange extract

1 teaspoon liquid stevia
(orange flavored, if possible)

5 cups ice cubes

DIRECTIONS

1 Place all the ingredients in a blender and puree until smooth.

2 Pour into glasses, garnish with a lime slice and serve immediately.

PER SERVING: *Calories 202; Fat 0g; Cholesterol 0mg; Sodium 1mg; Carbohydrates 2g (Dietary Fiber 0g, Sugar Alcohol 0g); Net Carbohydrates 2.2g; Protein 0g.*

CLASSIFYING KETO-FRIENDLY ALCOHOLS

Generally speaking, most alcohol is okay to consume on keto: it's actually the mixers used in most cocktails that tend to be off-limits. A substantial number of mixed drinks use juice and pure sugar syrups to get their flavor. Our recipes avoid all these sugar-laden mixers so you can create fresh, delicious cocktails that are incredibly flavorful while also being low-carb. Consider the following, which are great keto-friendly alcohols. You can use your imagination to make some great keto dessert drinks:

- **Hard liquors:** You can drink quite a few hard liquors while following a keto diet. Vodka, tequila, gin, rum, whiskey, and brandy are a few examples of alcohol that have zero carbs. Of course, be careful what you add, because that's where the sugary danger often lies.

- **Dry wines:** Red wine, white wine, rose, and sparkling wine are all very low in carbs. Avoid sweet wines such as Riesling or Moscato, because they're high in sugars. Most wine labels will list the carb count, making it easy to keep track of what you are consuming.

- **Light beers:** Light beers have significantly fewer carbs than regular, full-bodied brew. You can even find some beers on the market today that have zero carbs. Check the labels and make sure you consume in moderation.

- **Seltzer:** Seltzer and sparkling water are both excellent cocktail mixers. They have flavor but no added sugars and add a pleasant fizz to your drinks.

- **Fresh citrus juice:** Rather than pour bottled cranberry or orange juice, opt for a freshly squeezed citrus juice that contains fewer carbs but has just as much, if not more flavor. Fresh juice still has carbs, so be sure to add just a splash to get the taste you need.

🍅 Classic Gin Fizz

PREP TIME: 5 MIN   COOK TIME: 0 MIN   YIELD: 2 SERVINGS

INGREDIENTS

2 fresh cucumber slices

2 small lime slices

2 fresh mint leaves

½ cup gin

⅓ cup lime juice

2 cups sparkling water

4 ice cubes

DIRECTIONS

1 Place two ice cubes in each glass. Add one cucumber slice, one mint leaf, and one lime slice (squeeze the lime slice before adding it to the glass to help release some of the juice) in each glass as well.

2 Divide the gin and lime juice between the glasses and then top with the sparkling water. Garnish with a mint leaf and enjoy immediately.

PER SERVING: *Calories 160; Fat 0g; Cholesterol 0mg; Sodium 2mg; Carbohydrates 4g (Dietary Fiber 0g, Sugar Alcohol 0g); Net Carbohydrates 4.1g; Protein 0g.*

⏱ Keto Long Island Iced Tea

PREP TIME: 5 MIN	COOK TIME: 0 MIN	YIELD: 1 SERVING

INGREDIENTS

½ ounce vodka

½ ounce gin

½ ounce tequila

½ ounce light rum

1 tablespoon lime juice

1 tablespoon lemon juice

10 drops orange-flavored liquid stevia

1 cup ice

½ cup sugar-free cola

DIRECTIONS

1 Pour all the ingredients, except the cola, over ice into a cocktail shaker, cover, and shake for 30 seconds.

2 Pour the entire mixture into a large glass and top with the cola. Garnish with a small lemon slice and serve immediately.

PER SERVING: *Calories 141; Fat 0g; Cholesterol 0mg; Sodium 13mg; Carbohydrates 2g (Dietary Fiber 0g, Sugar Alcohol 0g); Net Carbohydrates 2.2g; Protein 0g.*

MAKING BIG BATCHES

You can make many of the cocktails in this chapter into large pitchers, which are perfect for parties. You can premeasure and premix all the alcohol, fresh juices, extracts, and sweeteners. We recommend adding the ice and the seltzers at the end if the recipe calls for these ingredients. Doing so keeps your premade cocktails from getting watered down and prevents the carbonated ingredients from going flat. Make a big batch and throw a party. No one will ever know the drinks are low-carb; they'll just know how great everything tastes.

Frozen Mudslide

PREP TIME: 5 MIN	COOK TIME: 0 MIN	YIELD: 2 SERVINGS

INGREDIENTS

¼ cup vodka

½ teaspoon vanilla extract

¼ cup heavy whipping cream

½ cup brewed coffee, cold

⅓ cup sugar-free Torani Irish cream coffee syrup

2 cups ice

2 tablespoons sugar-free chocolate syrup

DIRECTIONS

1 Place all the ingredients in a blender and puree until smooth.

2 Prepare two glasses with about 1 tablespoon of sugar-free chocolate syrup (Hershey's sugar-free chocolate syrup will work), dipping the rim of the glass in the syrup and letting it drip down the inside of the glass.

3 Pour into glasses and serve immediately.

PER SERVING: *Calories 170; Fat 11g; Cholesterol 41mg; Sodium 13mg; Carbohydrates 1g (Dietary Fiber 0g, Sugar Alcohol 0g); Net Carbohydrates 1g; Protein 1g.*

🍅 Blueberry Cosmopolitan

INGREDIENTS

3 ounces vodka

1 ounce lime juice

1 cup ice

5 drops orange-flavored liquid stevia

¼ cup fresh blueberries

DIRECTIONS

1 Place the blueberries and lime juice in a blender and puree until smooth.

2 Pour the blueberry mixture into a cocktail shaker over ice, and add vodka and stevia drops.

3 Cover the shaker and shake for 30 seconds. Strain into a martini glass, garnish with a small lime slice and single blueberry, and enjoy.

PER SERVING: *Calories 221; Fat 0g; Cholesterol 0mg; Sodium 2mg; Carbohydrates 8g (Dietary Fiber 1g, Sugar Alcohol 0g); Net Carbohydrates 6.7g; Protein 0g.*

🍅 Cranberry Lemon Spritzer

PREP TIME:10 MIN	COOK TIME: 0 MIN	YIELD: 2 SERVINGS

INGREDIENTS

½ cup fresh cranberries

1 tablespoon powdered erythritol

3 ounces vodka

2 tablespoons lemon juice

½ cup sparkling water

3 ice cubes

DIRECTIONS

1 Place the cranberries, powdered erythritol, vodka, and lemon juice in a blender and puree until smooth. Pass the mixture through a strainer to remove any cranberry seeds or skin.

2 Pour the strained cranberry mix into a tall glass with the ice cubes.

3 Top with the sparkling water and stir gently to combine. Garnish with a single whole cranberry and enjoy.

PER SERVING: *Calories 111; Fat 0g; Cholesterol 0mg; Sodium 1mg; Carbohydrates 10g (Dietary Fiber 2g, Sugar Alcohol 6g); Net Carbohydrates 2.8g; Protein 0g.*

Shaking Up Some Martinis

Do you like your drink shaken, not stirred? Well then we have some delicious keto drinks for you. If you have ever wondered why bartenders shake drinks before they serve them, we have the answer for you. At the very least, shaking a drink in a cocktail shaker with some ice will chill the drink thoroughly. You can then pour it into a glass, without the clunky ice cubes that water drinks down, and enjoy a crisp and cool beverage.

Shaking drinks also helps blend the flavors and gives the drink a little aeration. A nice frothy top may be the result as well. Try your hand at shaking some martinis with the recipes in this section. Give your shake a little flair so that you're mixing like a true, experienced mixologist.

⏱ Strawberry Lime Martini

PREP TIME: 2 MIN | **COOK TIME: 0 MIN** | **YIELD: 1 SERVING**

INGREDIENTS

¼ cup chopped strawberries

2 tablespoons lime juice

2 ounces vodka

½ cup ice

5 drops liquid stevia

DIRECTIONS

1 Puree the strawberries and lime juice in a blender until smooth.

2 Pour the pureed strawberries, vodka, and stevia over ice in a cocktail shaker, cover, and shake.

3 Strain into a martini glass, garnish with a small lime slice and enjoy.

PER SERVING: *Calories 146; Fat 0g; Cholesterol 0mg; Sodium 1mg; Carbohydrates 4g (Dietary Fiber 1g, Sugar Alcohol 0g); Net Carbohydrates 3.6g; Protein 0g.*

🍅 Chocolate Latte Martini

PREP TIME: 2 MIN	COOK TIME: 0 MIN	YIELD: 2 SERVINGS

INGREDIENTS

⅓ cup vodka

¼ teaspoon vanilla extract

1 teaspoon cocoa powder

8 drops chocolate-flavored stevia drops

1 tablespoon heavy whipping cream

1 ounce brewed espresso

1 cup ice

DIRECTIONS

1 Brew the espresso and add the cocoa powder to the warm espresso. Stir to dissolve.

2 Add the heavy whipping cream to the espresso mix and stir to help the espresso cool completely.

3 Add all the ingredients (including the espresso cream) to a cocktail shaker, cover and shake for 30 seconds.

4 Pour into two martini glasses, dust with a little extra unsweetened cocoa powder as a garnish and serve.

PER SERVING: *Calories 116; Fat 3g; Cholesterol 10mg; Sodium 5mg; Carbohydrates 1g (Dietary Fiber 0g, Sugar Alcohol 0g); Net Carbohydrates .7g; Protein 0g.*

3

Keto Desserts for Holidays and Special Occasions

IN THIS PART . . .

Show your low-carb love with these keto-approved sweets for Valentine's Day.

Scare the neighborhood by eliminating carbohydrates from your Halloween celebrations.

Give thanks for all the low-carb options you can load the table with on Thanksgiving.

Crack some eggs and the Easter bunny will be sure to show up for these delicious keto desserts.

Chase the cold gloominess of winter away with sweets that are sure to warm you to your soul.

Celebrate fresh beginnings by ushering in the New Year without breaking your macros.

Chapter **13**

Showing Your Loved Ones How You Feel: Keto Valentine's Day Desserts

Valentine's Day is the perfect day to make some delicious treats for your loved ones. Finding a delicious keto treat to enjoy on Valentine's Day can be difficult, but this isn't the day to hand your significant other a bowl of salad. You can stay on track with your macros while also pleasing those who aren't on keto. The recipes in this chapter are so tasty and sweet that no one will ever suspect that they're low-carb too.

Emphasizing Nutrition on Valentine's Day

Valentine's Day has long been a day of indulgence. It revolves around rich chocolate and pure decadence. Not many people think about nutrition on a holiday like this. However, if you're on keto, sticking to low-carb foods every day of the year is essential to help you stay in ketosis. Luckily, dark unsweetened chocolate, strawberries, and raspberries are all Valentine's Day icons and happen to be keto-friendly. Each of those ingredients also has impressive health benefits, allowing you to feel good about your holiday desserts.

High-quality dark chocolate is full of fiber, iron, and other beneficial minerals. It's a great source of natural antioxidants and has more than almost any other food in the world. Dark chocolate has been shown to help lower blood pressure and LDL cholesterol while protecting your skin from damaging UVB rays. The following recipes are mostly decadent desserts, many with dark chocolate.

Red Velvet Doughnuts

| PREP TIME: 25 MIN | COOK TIME: 20 MIN | YIELD: 12 DOUGHNUTS |

INGREDIENTS

2 cups almond flour, finely ground

½ cup granular erythritol

¼ cup sugar-free unflavored whey protein powder

¼ cup unsweetened cocoa powder

1 teaspoon xanthan gum

½ teaspoon baking soda

2 teaspoons baking powder

½ teaspoon salt

¾ cup plain Greek yogurt

¼ cup coconut oil, melted

3 eggs, room temperature

½ teaspoon vanilla extract

¼ cup heavy whipping cream

10 drops red gel food coloring

DIRECTIONS

1 Preheat the oven to 325 degrees F and grease two, six-cavity doughnut pans with cooking spray. These larger doughnut pans work better to get 12 large doughnuts.

2 Combine all the dry ingredients in a large bowl and whisk together. In a separate large bowl, beat together the yogurt, coconut oil, eggs, and vanilla extract until nicely combined. Add half the dry ingredients into the bowl with the wets and blend until smooth. Add the heavy whipping cream and beat again. Add the remaining dry ingredients and blend well. Add the red food coloring and mix until the color is all uniform.

3 Scoop the batter into the prepared doughnut pan and place in the preheated oven.

4 Bake for about 30 minutes or until the doughnuts are nice and firm. Remove from the oven and cool for about 5 minutes before flipping the doughnuts out of the pan onto a wire rack to cool completely. Store doughnuts in an airtight container for four to five days.

PER SERVING: *Calories 422; Fat 21g; Cholesterol 108mg; Sodium 439mg; Carbohydrates 19g (Dietary Fiber 5g, Sugar Alcohol 8g); Net Carbohydrates 5.3g; Protein 50g.*

COLORING YOUR FOOD RED

In addition to being all about chocolate, Valentine's Day is also known for bright red and pink colors. The majority of food colorings that you find in the grocery store are keto-approved, containing either no carbs or a very insignificant amount. When dying your baked goods, opt for a gel food coloring that is thick and requires less dye to get the color you want. You can also choose to make your own red food coloring by simmering chopped beets in water. Boil the mixture until the beets are fork-tender and the water is deep red. Store in the fridge until you're ready to use the dye. Just remember, you'll need a lot of the beet dye to get a bright, Valentine's Day red!

Peanut Butter Chocolate Hearts

INGREDIENTS

2 cups peanut butter, smooth, no sugar added

½ cup powdered erythritol

1 cup coconut flour

1 cup melted unsweetened chocolate chips

DIRECTIONS

1 Line a flat sheet tray with a piece of parchment paper and set aside.

2 Blend the peanut butter, powdered erythritol, and coconut flour in a large bowl until the batter is thick but smooth.

3 Divide the batter into 20 evenly sized balls and place on your prepared sheet tray. Shape each ball into a heart using your hands. Place the hearts in the freezer while your chocolate melts.

4 Melt the chocolate chips over a double boiler, stirring until smooth. All you need to melt chocolate over a double boiler is a small pot with about 2 cups of water in it. Bring the water to a boil and place a heatproof bowl on top of the pot. Make sure the bowl doesn't touch the boiling water. Add the unsweetened chocolate chips to the bowl and let the heat from the boiling water melt the chocolate. Stir occasionally to prevent the chocolate from burning.

5 Remove the hearts from the freezer, dipping each one into the melted chocolate, coating completely, and returning it to the tray. Dip all the hearts, let the chocolate cool, and then enjoy.

PER SERVING: *Calories 183; Fat 13g; Cholesterol 0mg; Sodium 18mg; Carbohydrates 17g (Dietary Fiber 6g, Sugar Alcohol 7g); Net Carbohydrates 5g; Protein 7g.*

Orange Chocolate Fat Bombs

PREP TIME: 10 MIN | COOK TIME: 1 MIN | YIELD: 10 FAT BOMBS

INGREDIENTS

1 cup cocoa powder, unsweetened

¼ cup melted coconut oil

5 tablespoons powdered erythritol

½ teaspoon orange extract

¼ teaspoon salt

1 tablespoon water

DIRECTIONS

1 In a large mixing bowl, combine all the ingredients together until a stiff, uniform batter has formed. If the mix is a little crumbly, add another tablespoon of water and blend until the dough comes together.

2 Scoop into 10 equally sized fat bombs, rolling the balls with your hands until smooth.

3 Store in an airtight container in the fridge for up to one week.

PER SERVING: *Calories 67; Fat 7g; Cholesterol 11mg; Sodium 52mg; Carbohydrates 11g (Dietary Fiber 3g, Sugar Alcohol 6g); Net Carbohydrates 1.8g; Protein 2g.*

NOTE: Fat bombs are similar to a granola bar, but they're more suitable for the keto diet. Fat bombs are very high in fats and low in carbs, and they can give you a great boost of energy in the middle of the day by providing your body with some long-lasting fuel (fats). One small fat bomb is a perfect snack or, in this case, a wonderful dessert that can satisfy your need for something sweet while sticking to your keto diet.

Dark Chocolate Fudge

| PREP TIME: 15 MIN | COOK TIME: 5 MIN | YIELD: 12 PIECES OF FUDGE |

INGREDIENTS

1 cup heavy whipping cream

⅓ cup granular erythritol

1 teaspoon vanilla extract

2 tablespoons butter

¼ teaspoon sea salt

1 cup dark chocolate chips, unsweetened

¼ cup chopped walnuts

DIRECTIONS

1 Place the heavy whipping cream, granular erythritol, vanilla extract, and the butter in a small saucepan. Heat over medium high heat, stirring frequently. Cook for 5 minutes.

2 Remove the pan from the heat and add the dark chocolate chips and salt and stir well until the chocolate is completely melted and blended into the heavy whipping cream mix. Pour the chocolate mix into a parchment-lined loaf pan and spread evenly.

3 Sprinkle the top of the fudge with the chopped walnuts and then place in the fridge for 1 hour to cool.

4 Slice into 12 pieces and enjoy. Store in an airtight container for up to two weeks.

PER SERVING: *Calories 152; Fat 15g; Cholesterol 32mg; Sodium 50mg; Carbohydrates 15g (Dietary Fiber 4g, Sugar Alcohol 8g); Net Carbohydrates 2.8g; Protein 2g.*

NOTE: In Step 1, the mixture should be thick, resembling sweetened condensed milk.

Getting Fruity with Your Valentine's Day Treats

Adding raspberries and strawberries is a great way to give your Valentine's Day the right color and to add some natural sweetness. Check out how these two keto-friendly fruits can highlight your Valentine's Day:

» **Raspberries:** Raspberries are naturally low in sugar but still taste sweet, making them a great addition to keto recipes. They're rich in antioxidants and can help prevent signs of aging while warding off diseases like cancer by preventing cancerous cells from spreading. Raspberries are also high in fiber, and eating them can promote a healthy gut.

» **Strawberries:** Strawberries contain a lot of water and very few carbs. They also have high quantities of fiber, as well as lots of vitamins and minerals such as vitamin C, manganese, and potassium. Strawberries are also a hallmark of Valentine's Day, and many holiday desserts revolve around this delicious, keto-approved fruit.

☕ Chocolate-Covered Strawberries

PREP TIME: 10 MIN	COOK TIME: 1 MIN	YIELD: 14 STRAWBERRIES

INGREDIENTS

½ cup unsweetened dark chocolate chips

2 tablespoons coconut oil

14 whole strawberries, stems on

DIRECTIONS

1 Set up a double boiler using a small pot with about 2 cups of water. Bring the water to a boil and place a heatproof bowl on top of the pot, making sure the bowl doesn't touch the boiling water. Place the chocolate chips and coconut oil in the bowl and heat until melted completely (about 3 to 5 minutes). Stir occasionally to blend the ingredients together and make smooth. Prepare a sheet tray with a piece of parchment.

2 Dip the strawberries, one at a time, in the melted chocolate. Let the dipped strawberries drip over the chocolate bowl briefly and then place them on the prepared sheet tray to chill. If you start to run low on chocolate as you dip each berry, pour the chocolate into a smaller container, making it a little deeper for dipping. You can also spoon the melted chocolate over the berry.

3 Store in the fridge and enjoy once the chocolate hardens.

PER SERVING: *Calories 42; Fat 4g; Cholesterol 0mg; Sodium 1mg; Carbohydrates 5g (Dietary Fiber 2g, Sugar Alcohol 1g); Net Carbohydrates 1.5g; Protein .5g.*

VARY IT: Dip the strawberries in unsweetened toasted coconut or toasted chopped nuts for extra flavor.

Dark Chocolate Raspberry Cheesecake

PREP TIME: 10 MIN	COOK TIME: 50–60 MIN	YIELD: 12 SERVINGS

INGREDIENTS

1½ cups finely ground almond flour

2½ tablespoons granular erythritol

1 tablespoon unsweetened cocoa powder

4 tablespoons butter, melted

1 pound cream cheese, softened

½ cup granular erythritol

2 eggs

½ teaspoon vanilla extract

¼ cup dark chocolate chips, unsweetened

2 tablespoons melted butter

1 cup fresh raspberries

DIRECTIONS

1 Preheat the oven to 350 degrees F and grease a 9-inch spring-form pan with baking spray or coconut oil. Set the prepared pan aside.

2 In a medium bowl, combine the almond flour, 2½ tablespoons granular erythritol, unsweetened cocoa powder, and 4 table-spoons melted butter. Stir together well and then use your hands to scoop the mix into the prepared pan. Press down, covering the bottom of the pan evenly with the crust. Place a piece of foil over the crust and add pie weights on top of the foil. Bake the crust for 10 minutes and then set aside to cool, removing the weights and the foil.

3 Lower the oven heat to 300 degrees F.

4 In a medium mixing bowl, beat the cream cheese and ½ cup granular erythritol until light and fluffy. Add the eggs and vanilla extract and stir until just combined.

5 In a separate small bowl, mix the chocolate chips and butter and melt in the microwave. Stir the chocolate and butter to combine and then pour into the cream cheese mix, stirring well. Fold in the fresh raspberries, stirring only a few times so as not to crush the berries. Pour the filling over the cheesecake crust and then spread so the cake is level.

6 Bake the cheesecake for 40 to 50 minutes or until set in the center. Allow the cheesecake to cool completely in the pan and then remove the springform pan sides. Wrap the cake gently and cool in the fridge for several hours to help the cake firm. Slice and serve. Wrap any extra cheesecake in plastic wrap and store in the fridge for up to one week.

PER SERVING: *Calories 294; Fat 28g; Cholesterol 92mg; Sodium 151mg; Carbohydrates 19g (Dietary Fiber 3g, Sugar Alcohol 11g); Net Carbohydrates 4g; Protein 7g.*

TIP: You can use frozen raspberries during off-season. Just don't thaw them.

Raspberry Gummy Bears

INGREDIENTS

5 tablespoons gelatin powder

½ cup water

2 cups coconut milk, canned, full fat

½ cup water

1 cup pureed raspberries

1 teaspoon granular erythritol

DIRECTIONS

1 Mix the gelatin with ½ cup of water and let sit for 5 minutes. Add to a small saucepan and heat over low heat to melt.

2 Add the coconut milk, remaining water, and raspberry puree to the saucepan and heat over medium heat, whisking until the mixture is smooth and warm. Add the granular erythritol and whisk again. As soon as the mix begins to steam, turn off the heat.

3 Use an eyedropper to fill the gummy bear mold with the mixture.

4 Place the gummy bear trays in the fridge to set completely (this takes about an hour, depending on the size of your gummy bear mold).

5 Pop the gummy bears out of the tray and enjoy. Store in an airtight container for up to a week.

PER SERVING: *Calories 92; Fat 8g; Cholesterol 0mg; Sodium 11mg; Carbohydrates 3g (Dietary Fiber 1g, Sugar Alcohol 0g); Net Carbohydrates 1.9g; Protein 3g.*

NOTE: If you don't have a gummy bear mold or other small silicone mold, pour the mixture into a shallow glass container and let chill. Slice the gummies into squares and enjoy.

NOTE: Using an eyedropper allows you to get the perfect amount of mix into each gummy bear cavity, giving each bear its perfect shape.

Strawberry Cheesecake Bites

PREP TIME: 10 MIN	COOK TIME: 0 MIN	YIELD: 12 BITES

INGREDIENTS

1 cup diced strawberries

1 teaspoon vanilla extract

¼ cup coconut oil, melted

⅛ teaspoon salt

6 ounces cream cheese, softened

DIRECTIONS

1 Line a muffin tin with paper cupcake liners and set aside.

2 Place the strawberries in a blender or food processor and puree until smooth. Add the remaining ingredients and puree again until the batter is completely smooth and blended. Pour the strawberry cheesecake mix into the prepared tray, filling each muffin cup about a quarter full.

3 Place the tray in the freezer and freeze for about 2 hours or until completely solid. Enjoy right away or store in an airtight container in the freezer for up to a month.

PER SERVING: *Calories 93; Fat 9g; Cholesterol 16mg; Sodium 73mg; Carbohydrates 1.7g (Dietary Fiber .3g); Net Carbohydrates 1.4g; Protein 1g.*

🍓 Strawberry Shortcakes

PREP TIME: 10 MIN	COOK TIME: 20 MIN	YIELD: 12 SHORTCAKES

INGREDIENTS

3 cups almond flour, finely ground

½ cup granular erythritol

1 teaspoon salt

½ teaspoon baking soda

3 eggs, room temperature

¾ cup heavy whipping cream

1 teaspoon vanilla extract

½ teaspoon liquid stevia drops

3 cups diced strawberries

2 tablespoons powdered erythritol

¼ teaspoon vanilla extract

1 cup heavy whipping cream

2 tablespoons powdered erythritol

¼ teaspoon vanilla extract

DIRECTIONS

1 Preheat the oven to 350 degrees F and prepare a sheet tray with a piece of parchment paper.

2 Place the almond flour, granular erythritol, salt, and baking soda in a large bowl. Mix to combine. Add the eggs, ¾ cup heavy whipping cream, 1 teaspoon vanilla extract, and liquid stevia to the dry ingredients and stir until a thick, sticky batter has formed.

3 Scoop the batter onto the prepared sheet tray, making 12 equal shortcakes. Bake in the preheated oven for 20 minutes or until golden brown. Remove from the oven and cool.

4 Place the strawberries, 2 tablespoons powdered erythritol, and ¼ teaspoon vanilla extract in a bowl and toss together. Set aside. In a new medium bowl, combine the 1 cup heavy whipping cream, 2 tablespoons powdered erythritol, and remaining ¼ teaspoon vanilla extract. Whisk together until stiff peaks form.

5 To assemble the shortcakes, slice each mini cake in half and put on a plate. Add a scoop of the strawberries to the middle of the cake and then top with the prepared whipped cream. Serve immediately. If you're waiting to enjoy these shortcakes until a later time, store the biscuits at room temperature, wrapped tightly in plastic wrap. Keep the strawberries and whipped cream in the fridge for up to one day.

PER SERVING: *Calories 317; Fat 28g; Cholesterol 101mg; Sodium 251mg; Carbohydrates 22g (Dietary Fiber 4g, Sugar Alcohol 12g); Net Carbohydrates 5.9g; Protein 9g.*

Chapter **14**

Getting Spooky with Halloween Keto Fun

Halloween is a time when black and orange reign and anything spooky or creepy is acceptable. It may be the only time of year when you can create scary-looking food and people will get excited about it. In addition to the fun side of Halloween, rich fall flavors are also in style. That means lots of pumpkin and plenty of cinnamon in many dishes, drinks, and especially desserts. This chapter gives you a nice mix of fun, spooky treats alongside several classic pumpkin tastes.

Discovering the Health Benefits of Pumpkin

The fact that pumpkin is in season around Halloween is perfect. In addition to perfect color coordination with the holiday, pumpkin is also quite healthy. This squash family member is high in vitamin A and low in calories, and it's an excellent source of many other vitamins and minerals. Vitamins A and C boost your immune system, whereas antioxidants reduce your risk of chronic disease. In fact, pumpkin is so nutrient-dense that it can help promote weight loss by satiating your hunger after eating a relatively small amount of pumpkin-based foods. Pumpkin has some carbohydrates, but very few, and as long as you stay within your macros, you'll be fine. Enjoy these tasty pumpkin recipes and reap the benefits of healthy baking.

Pumpkin Cookies

PREP TIME: 5 MIN	COOK TIME: 12 MIN	YIELD: 18 COOKIES

INGREDIENTS

1 cup butter, softened

⅔ cup granular erythritol

1 egg, room temperature

1 teaspoon vanilla extract

½ cup pumpkin puree

2 cups almond flour

½ cup coconut flour

1½ teaspoons pumpkin pie spice

1 teaspoon baking powder

½ teaspoon xanthan gum

DIRECTIONS

1 Preheat your oven to 350 degrees F and prepare a cookie sheet with parchment paper or a silicone mat.

2 Use an electric mixer to beat the butter and erythritol until light and creamy. Add the egg, vanilla extract, and pumpkin puree to the butter mix and blend well until fully combined. Add the almond flour, coconut flour, pumpkin pie spice, baking powder, and xanthan gum to the bowl and stir to form a smooth batter.

3 Scoop the cookies into 1-inch balls and place on the prepared cookie sheet.

4 Bake for 12 minutes or until the edges of the cookies begin to brown. Remove the tray from the oven, cool on a wire rack, and enjoy. Store the cookies in an airtight container at room temperature for up to one week.

PER SERVING: *Calories 184; Fat 17g; Cholesterol 39mg; Sodium 34mg; Carbohydrates 12g (Dietary Fiber 3g, Sugar Alcohol 7g); Net Carbohydrates 2.2g; Protein 4g.*

FINDING THE PERFECT PUMPKIN PUREE

When baking fall-inspired recipes, you'll see a lot of recipes call for pumpkin puree. At the grocery store, you may find various kinds of canned pumpkin puree. You may also wonder if you should use real pumpkin and make your own. So which kind of pumpkin is really best for baking?

If you opt to use canned pumpkin puree, make sure it's 100 percent pumpkin with nothing else added into the mix. Grocery stores tend to carry pumpkin pie filling in similar cans to the pure puree. Make sure you don't grab a pumpkin pie puree because it contains added spices and sugars (not good for the keto diet). Pure pumpkin puree is exactly what you're looking for.

Roasting and pureeing your own pumpkin is definitely a viable option. Cut a small pumpkin into quarters, remove the seeds, drizzle with some olive oil, and then roast in a 450 degree oven for about 40 to 60 minutes (depending on the size of your pumpkin). Scoop the flesh away from the skin of the pumpkin and puree it in a blender or food processor until smooth. Homemade puree works great in recipes; however, it does take a significant amount of effort and truly doesn't affect the taste of your baked goods.

Chocolate Chip Pumpkin Bars

PREP TIME: 10 MIN	COOK TIME: 20 MIN	YIELD: 16 BARS

INGREDIENTS

¼ cup butter

2 ounces cream cheese

1 cup pumpkin puree

2 eggs, room temperature

1 teaspoon vanilla extract

1 cup finely ground almond flour

⅔ cup granular erythritol

2 teaspoons baking powder

1 teaspoon pumpkin pie spice

¼ teaspoon sea salt

1 cup finely chopped unsweetened chocolate

DIRECTIONS

1 Preheat the oven to 350 degrees F and line a 9x9-inch pan with parchment paper.

2 Place the butter and cream cheese in a microwave-safe bowl and heat for about 30 seconds to melt. Add the melted cream cheese and butter mixture with pumpkin puree, eggs, and vanilla extract in a large bowl and blend well. Add the almond flour, granular erythritol, baking powder, pumpkin pie spice, and sea salt to the bowl and mix to form a smooth batter. Fold the chopped chocolate into the batter by hand and then scoop into the prepared pan.

3 Spread the batter until even and flat and then bake for 25 minutes or until it's completely set in the center. Remove from the oven, let cool completely in the pan, and then slice and serve. Store in the refrigerator, wrapped well, for up to one week.

PER SERVING: *Calories 132; Fat 12g; Cholesterol 38mg; Sodium 213mg; Carbohydrates 18g (Dietary Fiber 4g, Sugar Alcohol 10g); Net Carbohydrates 3g; Protein 4g.*

Having Fun with Halloween Baking

Halloween is a great time to let your inner decorator take over. You can quickly make a basic keto dessert into something festive with a bit of imagination and a little food coloring. The following section gives you some great ideas. Here are some additional ways you can make your desserts extra exciting this Halloween:

» **Gravestone cookies:** Make the Cinnamon "Sugar" Cookies from Chapter 7 and bake the cookies in gravestone shapes (round the top of a rectangle). Spread melted, unsweetened dark chocolate and then use softened cream cheese to pipe "RIP" on each one. Gravestones complete!

» **Pumpkin fat bombs:** Make some pumpkin-flavored fat bombs (refer to Chapter 13) and dye them orange for a fun Halloween twist. You can shape them into mini pumpkins, using a single dark chocolate chip as the stem. You can share these treats with everyone.

» **Spooky ice cubes:** Liven up your Halloween drinks by making some spooky ice cubes. Place a plastic spider in each cavity of an ice cube tray and then fill with water. Use the frozen spider cubes for any drink.

» **Ghost cupcakes:** Make the following Spider Web Cupcakes recipe, but frost them with white icing. Use two unsweetened dark chocolate chips for eyes and you have ghost cupcakes!

» **Witch fingers:** Use the following Candy Corn Cookies recipe, but dye all the batter green instead. Pipe small logs and place a sliced almond at the top of each cookie before baking. You've just created Witch Finger cookies!

🍅 Candy Corn Cookies

INGREDIENTS

2 cups almond flour, finely ground

⅓ cup granular erythritol

½ cup butter, softened

1 egg

1 teaspoon vanilla extract

Orange food coloring, about 4–5 drops

Yellow food coloring, about 4–5 drops

DIRECTIONS

1 Place the almond flour and granular erythritol in a bowl and mix together. Add the softened butter and use your hands to blend the butter into the dry ingredients until fine crumbles form. Add the egg and vanilla extract and knead into a soft dough.

2 Divide the dough into three equal sections and place in three separate bowls.

3 Add some orange food coloring to one bowl and blend the dough until uniform in color. Add some yellow food coloring to a separate bowl and blend the dough until it's evenly yellow.

4 Roll each color of dough into a log about 1½ inches wide. Press the logs together with the white dough at the bottom, orange in the middle and yellow dough at the top. Press gently to flatten and press together. You should have a long, striped strip of dough about 1 inch high and around 16 inches long.

5 Place a piece of parchment paper on top of the dough and roll gently to flatten the dough, pressing the colors together and making one quarter-inch thick strip of cookie dough on the tray. Place in the freezer for 20 minutes to firm.

6 Preheat your oven to 300 degrees F.

7 Remove the dough from the freezer and take the top piece of parchment paper off the dough. Cut the dough into triangles to look like candy corn. Place the cookies on a new, parchment-lined cookie sheet leaving about 1 inch of space between each cookie.

8 Bake for about 20 minutes or until the edges begin to turn golden brown. Remove from the tray, cool, and then enjoy. Store in an airtight container at room temperature for up to one week.

PER SERVING: *Calories 92; Fat 9g; Cholesterol 19mg; Sodium 4mg; Carbohydrates 5g (Dietary Fiber 1g, Sugar Alcohol 3g); Net Carbohydrates 1g; Protein 2g.*

🍅 Spider Web Cupcakes

PREP TIME: 40 MIN | COOK TIME: 30 MIN | YIELD: 16 CUPCAKES

INGREDIENTS

1¼ cups almond flour, finely ground

⅓ cup unflavored sugar-free whey protein powder

⅔ cup powdered erythritol

1 teaspoon ground cinnamon

1 teaspoon baking soda

2 teaspoons apple cider vinegar

¼ cup butter, melted

8 eggs

1 cup pumpkin puree

½ cup heavy whipping cream

15 drops liquid stevia

½ cup butter, softened

1 cup softened cream cheese

½ cup powdered erythritol

½ teaspoon vanilla extract

¼ teaspoon sea salt

Black gel food coloring

DIRECTIONS

1 Preheat your oven to 350 degrees F and prepare a muffin tray by placing a paper cupcake liner in each cavity. Set aside.

2 Place the almond flour, protein powder, ⅔ cup powdered erythritol, cinnamon, and baking soda in a large bowl. Whisk together. In a separate bowl, blend the apple cider vinegar, melted butter, eggs, pumpkin puree, heavy whipping cream, and liquid stevia together until smooth. Mix the dry ingredients together with the wet mixture and blend until smooth.

3 Scoop the batter into the prepared muffin cups and bake in the preheated oven for 30 minutes or until the tops are firm to the touch (start checking the cupcakes after about 20 minutes) and then remove them and let them cool completely on a wire rack while you make the frosting.

4 To make the frosting, beat the butter, cream cheese, and ½ cup powdered erythritol in a bowl. Whip until light and fluffy before adding the vanilla extract and salt. Stir well. Place a small amount of the frosting in a separate bowl, add a few drops of the black food coloring, and mix until evenly colored. Place the black food coloring in a piping bag with a very small, straight tip.

5 Spread the white frosting on the top of each cupcake, spreading as smooth as possible. Pipe the black frosting onto the cupcake, making a spiral.

6 Take a toothpick and start at the center of the cupcake and drag the toothpick outward, making a spider web effect in the black and white frosting. Repeat with all the cupcakes.

PER SERVING: *Calories 246; Fat 23g; Cholesterol 155mg; Sodium 208mg; Carbohydrates 18g (Dietary Fiber 2g, Sugar Alcohol 14g); Net Carbohydrates 2.6g; Protein 6g.*

Mummy Cookies

PREP TIME: 20 MIN	COOK TIME: 12 MIN	YIELD: 12 COOKIES

INGREDIENTS

½ cup almond flour, finely ground

½ cup coconut flour

¼ cup granular erythritol

2 eggs, room temperature

4 tablespoons butter, softened

1 teaspoon vanilla extract

½ cup softened cream cheese

1 ounce heavy whipping cream

1 tablespoon powdered erythritol

1 tablespoon dark chocolate chips

DIRECTIONS

1 Preheat your oven to 350 degrees F and line a cookie sheet with parchment paper or a silicone mat.

2 Combine the almond flour, coconut flour, and granular erythritol in a large bowl and mix well. Add the eggs, softened butter, and vanilla extract to the bowl and mix until a smooth batter forms.

3 Scoop the cookie dough into 12 equally sized balls and place on the prepared cookie sheet. Press the dough down to flatten slightly. Bake the cookies for 12 minutes or until the edges begin to turn golden brown. Remove from the oven and let the cookies cool completely on a wire rack.

4 To make the frosting, in a separate bowl whip the cream cheese, heavy whipping cream, and powdered erythritol together until smooth. Place the frosting in a piping bag with a small straight tip.

5 After the cookies have cooled, draw lines diagonally across the cookies, going back and forth with the icing like a mummy being wrapped. Place two chocolate chips near the top of the cookie to be the mummies eyes. Store the cookies in the fridge for up to one week after baking, wrapped in an airtight container.

PER SERVING: *Calories 127; Fat 11g; Cholesterol 24mg; Sodium 47mg; Carbohydrates 10g (Dietary Fiber 2g, Sugar Alcohol 6g); Net Carbohydrates 2g; Protein 3g.*

☺ Black and Orange Brownies

| PREP TIME: 15 MIN | COOK TIME: 30 MIN | YIELD: 10 BROWNIES |

INGREDIENTS

2 eggs, room temperature

½ cup coconut oil

1 teaspoon vanilla extract

¾ cup granular erythritol

½ cup almond flour

½ cup unsweetened cocoa powder

¼ teaspoon baking powder

½ teaspoon sea salt

1 cup cream cheese, softened

¼ cup powdered erythritol

1 egg

½ teaspoon vanilla extract

5 drops orange food coloring

DIRECTIONS

1 Preheat the oven to 350 degrees F and line a 9x9-inch pan with parchment paper.

2 In a medium bowl, combine the eggs, coconut oil, and vanilla extract until well blended. Add the granular erythritol, almond flour, cocoa powder, baking powder, and salt and stir to form a smooth batter. Scoop the batter into the prepared pan and spread to smooth evenly.

3 In a new bowl, beat the cream cheese, powdered erythritol, egg, and vanilla extract together. Once smooth, add the orange food coloring and stir again.

4 Spread the cream cheese mixture on top of the chocolate mix in the pan.

5 Bake in the preheated oven for 20 to 30 minutes or until a toothpick inserted in the center comes out cleanly. Cook slightly less for chewier brownies and longer for crunchy brownies. Let the brownies cool in the pan and then slice and serve.

PER SERVING: *Calories 238; Fat 24g; Cholesterol 89mg; Sodium 232mg; Carbohydrates 24g (Dietary Fiber 2g, Sugar Alcohol 19g); Net Carbohydrates 2g; Protein 5g.*

NOTE: In Step 4, it's okay if the cream cheese mixture and chocolate mix swirl together slightly but try to keep the two layers separate.

Chapter **15**

Making Keto Desserts for Thanksgiving

Thanksgiving is family time, but it's also an occasion for delicious dishes. In fact, the entire holiday revolves around food. That doesn't mean that you can ignore your macros and get off track, though. The good news: this chapter is chock-full of keto-friendly Thanksgiving dishes. There's no reason why your diet and your taste buds can't both be at the top of their games.

Embracing Pie at Thanksgiving

Pies tend to be the most common dessert at Thanksgiving, and they're often the default when someone is trying to pick out a sweet dish. Traditionally, pies are made with lots of white flour in the crust, with fillings that are also super sugary, which isn't very keto at all. However, missing out on pie would be an absolute travesty, which is why we developed these recipes in this section. You can also make slight modifications to the following pie favorites to make them more keto-friendly:

>> **Pumpkin pie:** Pumpkin pie became associated with Thanksgiving around the 19th century. This orange squash is native to the United States and comes into season in the early fall every year. This coincidence led to pumpkin becoming a holiday staple, which is good news for low-carb dieters like you. Add a bit of maple extract to your keto pumpkin pie to make it even more vibrant and delicious.

>> **Apple pie:** Apple pie is popular at Thanksgiving, in large part because apple season is around the same time, making apples abundant and delicious. The traditional recipe typically contains brown sugar, but you can easily replace this ingredient with golden erythritol to achieve that deep, rich flavor. Apples pair perfectly with an almond flour crust, creating a match made in keto heaven.

🍅 Pumpkin Mousse

PREP TIME: 15 MIN	COOK TIME: 0 MIN	YIELD: 6 SERVINGS

INGREDIENTS

1 15-ounce can pumpkin puree

1 teaspoon pumpkin pie spice

¼ teaspoon salt

1½ teaspoons vanilla extract

¾ cup heavy whipping cream

¼ cup granular erythritol

¼ cup heavy whipping cream

1 tablespoon granular erythritol

¼ teaspoon ground cinnamon

DIRECTIONS

1 In a large bowl, combine the pumpkin puree, pumpkin pie spice, salt, and vanilla extract. In a separate large bowl, whip the ¾ cup heavy whipping cream and ¼ cup granular erythritol until soft peaks form. Fold the pumpkin mix and the heavy whipping cream together gently until just combined.

2 Scoop the mousse into six serving cups.

3 Whip the remaining heavy whipping cream, granular erythritol, and cinnamon together and place a dollop of the whipped cream on top of each mousse cup. Serve immediately.

PER SERVING: *Calories 167; Fat 15g; Cholesterol 54mg; Sodium 116mg; Carbohydrates 18g (Dietary Fiber 2g, Sugar Alcohol 10g); Net Carbohydrates 5.4g; Protein 2g.*

NOTE: Pour this mousse into a pre-baked keto pie crust for a fantastic pumpkin mousse pie recipe.

🍅 Keto Chocolate Chip Cookie Pie

INGREDIENTS

1½ cups almond flour

¼ cup ground flaxseed

1 tablespoon golden erythritol

6 tablespoons melted butter

1 egg

½ cup almond flour

⅔ cup golden erythritol

¾ cup butter, melted

2 eggs, room temperature

1 cup unsweetened dark chocolate chips

DIRECTIONS

1 Preheat your oven to 325 degrees F.

2 In a large bowl, combine the 1½ cups almond flour, flaxseeds, 1 tablespoon golden erythritol, 6 tablespoons butter, and egg. Blend well and then pour the mix into a 9-inch pie pan. Press the mix into the bottom of the pan and up the sides.

3 Bake the crust in the preheated oven for 10 minutes and then remove from the oven and set aside.

4 In a large mixing bowl, mix the remaining almond flour and golden erythritol together. Add the butter and eggs and mix well. Fold in the dark chocolate chips and then pour the mix into the prepared pie pan.

5 Bake the pie for 55 minutes. Let the pie cool for at least 30 minutes before slicing and serving. Store this pie for four to five days at room temperature, wrapped well with plastic wrap.

PER SERVING: *Calories 245; Fat 24g; Cholesterol 85mg; Sodium 17mg; Carbohydrates 20g (Dietary Fiber 5g, Sugar Alcohol 13g); Net Carbohydrates 2.5g; Protein 5g.*

TIP: In Step 5, bake the pie until the pie has just a slight jiggle in the center.

TRYING BROWN SUGAR ALTERNATIVES

Thanksgiving ushers in cold weather and a corresponding desire for comfort foods. One way to make your keto baking warmer and richer, adding layers of deep flavor, is to choose a golden sweetener. Golden keto sweeteners are comparable in taste to brown sugar but usually contain no net carbs. Real brown sugar is definitely off-limits. Monk fruit and erythritol golden sweeteners are fairly common, and most can be used as a 1:1 replacement for brown sugar.

🍅 Pecan Pie

PREP TIME: 5 MIN   COOK TIME: 60 MIN   YIELD: 12 SERVINGS

INGREDIENTS

½ cup almond flour

¼ cup coconut flour

½ cup granular erythritol

1 teaspoon vanilla extract

1 egg

2 tablespoons butter

¾ cup butter

¾ cup powdered erythritol and monk fruit blend

1½ cups heavy whipping cream

1 teaspoon sea salt

1½ teaspoons vanilla extract

1 teaspoon maple extract (optional)

1 egg

2 cups chopped pecans

DIRECTIONS

1 Place the almond flour, coconut flour, ½ cup granular erythritol, 1 teaspoon vanilla extract, egg, and 2 tablespoons butter in a food processor. Blend until a smooth dough forms. Wrap the ball of dough and place in the fridge to chill for 30 minutes.

2 Preheat the oven to 375 degrees F. Place the dough between two pieces of parchment paper and roll into a 9-inch circle. Place the dough into an 8-inch tart pan, pushing the dough up the sides of the pan and making the crust as even as possible. Bake for 15 minutes.

3 Lower the oven heat to 350 degrees F. While the crust is baking, make the caramel for the pie. In a small saucepan, heat the butter and powdered erythritol and monk fruit blend. Stir to melt the sweetener and allow the mix to turn slightly golden, about 5 minutes. Slowly add the heavy whipping cream, stirring constantly. Add the salt and both extracts and then remove from the heat and let cool for about 10 minutes. The mix should still be warm but not hot.

4 Add the egg to the caramel sauce, whisking well. Pour the chopped pecans into the pie crust and then pour the caramel sauce over the nuts.

5 Place the pie in the oven and bake for 40 minutes or until the filling has set. If the pie starts to get too dark, lightly cover it with a piece of foil and continue baking until set. Cool the pie completely before slicing and serving. Store, wrapped well, in the refrigerator for up to one week.

PER SERVING: *Calories 277; Fat 28g; Cholesterol 84mg; Sodium 216mg; Carbohydrates 24g (Dietary Fiber 3g, Sugar Alcohol 20g); Net Carbohydrates 1.7g; Protein 4g.*

NOTE: In Step 3, after 15 minutes the crust won't be completely cooked, but it will finish cooking with the filling.

Adding Nuts to Your Thanksgiving Keto Desserts

Nuts find their way into desserts as the weather starts to get colder. Luckily, many kinds of nuts are great for keto. They not only fit well with the cold weather and seasonal traditions, but they're also an excellent match for low-carb macros. If you happen to be allergic to nuts, many of these recipes work well by simply eliminating the nut component. Assess each recipe and see whether the nuts are there for recipe integrity or just for taste; if they are purely for extra taste and texture, feel free to skip them.

Here are some nuts you can incorporate in your keto Thanksgiving recipes:

>> **Almonds:** Almonds have a nice crunch when baked and are full of flavor. You can find many kinds of almonds in the grocery store as well — sliced, chopped, or whole — giving you options for any recipe.

>> **Hazelnuts:** Hazelnuts are rich and decadent. They add a nice warm flavor to any dish and pair well with chocolate.

>> **Pecans:** Pecans are a Thanksgiving classic thanks to pecan pie. Pecans give desserts a delicious nutty taste while being nice and soft. They practically melt in your mouth.

>> **Walnuts:** When eaten alone, walnuts can have an almost drying texture and taste but, when paired with the right dessert, their amazing flavor really shines through.

Here are some of our favorite keto Thanksgiving recipes with nuts.

Pumpkin Crunch Cake

PREP TIME: 15 MIN | **COOK TIME: 55 MIN** | **YIELD: 10 SERVINGS**

INGREDIENTS

5 eggs, room temperature

1 cup pumpkin puree

½ cup powdered erythritol

1 tablespoon pumpkin pie spice

½ cup butter, melted

1 teaspoon vanilla extract

⅔ cup coconut flour

½ teaspoon sea salt

½ tablespoon baking powder

¼ cup cream cheese, softened

¾ tablespoon powdered erythritol

½ tablespoon heavy whipping cream

½ teaspoon vanilla extract

3 tablespoons butter, melted

⅓ cup chopped pecans

1½ tablespoons coconut flour

⅓ cup golden erythritol

1 teaspoon pumpkin pie spice

DIRECTIONS

1 Preheat your oven to 350 degrees F and prepare a rectangular baking pan by greasing the bottom and sides.

2 In a large bowl, beat the eggs, pumpkin puree, ½ cup powdered erythritol, and 1 tablespoon pumpkin pie spice until well mixed. Add the melted butter and 1 teaspoon vanilla extract to the bowl and stir well to combine.

3 Add the ⅔ cup coconut flour, ½ teaspoon salt, and ½ tablespoon baking powder and mix into a smooth batter. Pour the batter into the prepared baking pan.

4 In a new, clean bowl, combine the cream cheese, ¾ tablespoon powdered erythritol, heavy whipping cream, and ½ teaspoon vanilla extract until smooth. Spoon a few dollops of the cream cheese gently over the pumpkin batter in the pan, distributing it throughout the pan evenly. Use a knife to swirl the cream cheese into the pumpkin layer gently.

5 In a new bowl, mix 3 tablespoons melted butter, pecans, coconut flour, golden erythritol, and pumpkin pie spice. Mix until crumbly and then sprinkle over the top of the batter in the baking pan.

6 Bake for 25 to 30 minutes. Let cool for at least 20 minutes before slicing and serving.

PER SERVING: *Calories 257; Fat 23g; Cholesterol 147mg; Sodium 247mg; Carbohydrates 25g (Dietary Fiber 4g, Sugar Alcohol 17g); Net Carbohydrates 4g; Protein 6g.*

🍅 Almond Cheesecake

PREP TIME: 15 MIN	COOK TIME: 60 MIN	YIELD: 12 SERVINGS

INGREDIENTS

1½ cups almond flour, finely ground

¼ cup butter, melted

2 tablespoons granular erythritol

¾ tsp ground cinnamon

1½ cups cream cheese, room temperature

¼ cup butter, room temperature

1 cup powdered erythritol

3 eggs, room temperature

¾ cup sour cream

½ tablespoon almond extract

DIRECTIONS

1 Preheat your oven to 300 degrees F.

2 Grease a 9-inch, springform cake pan and place a round piece of parchment in the bottom of the pan. Wrap the outside of the pan with aluminum foil and then set the pan aside.

3 In a medium bowl, combine the almond flour, ¼ cup melted butter, 2 tablespoons granular erythritol, and cinnamon. Mix well and then pour into the prepared cake pan. Press firmly into the bottom and then set aside.

4 Beat the cream cheese and butter together until light and fluffy. Add the powdered erythritol to the bowl and beat to combine well. Add the eggs one at a time, scraping down the sides of the bowl after each addition. Add the sour cream and almond extract and stir until a smooth batter forms. Pour the batter into the prepared pan and then place the pan in a water bath.

5 Bake in the preheated oven for about 60 minutes. After 50 minutes, start checking to see whether the cheesecake has already set.

6 Remove the cheesecake from the oven and run a spatula around the edge of the pan to prevent the cake from sticking. Let the cheesecake cool completely before removing from the pan. Chill in the fridge before slicing and serving.

PER SERVING: *Calories 176; Fat 17g; Cholesterol 91mg; Sodium 61mg; Carbohydrates 20g (Dietary Fiber 1g, Sugar Alcohol 18g); Net Carbohydrates 1.4g; Protein 4g.*

NOTE: In Step 5, the cheesecake is set when the center slightly jiggles but is firm around the edges.

Chocolate Pecan Bars

PREP TIME: 10 MIN	COOK TIME: 30 MIN	YIELD: 12 BARS

INGREDIENTS

1 cup coconut flour

¼ cup powdered erythritol

⅓ cup coconut oil

1–2 tablespoons water

½ cup coconut oil

⅔ cup granular erythritol

½ teaspoon vanilla extract

¼ teaspoon sea salt

2 cups chopped pecans

½ cup dark chocolate chips, unsweetened

DIRECTIONS

1 Preheat your oven to 350 degrees F and prepare an 8x8-inch cake pan with a piece of parchment in the bottom.

2 In a medium mixing bowl, combine the coconut flour, powdered erythritol, and ⅓ cup coconut oil. Blend until crumbly. If the mix is too dry, add 1 to 2 tablespoons water.

3 Press the mix into the prepared pan to make a crust and then bake in the oven for 15 minutes or until the top begins to turn golden brown.

4 Add ½ cup coconut oil, granular erythritol, vanilla extract, and sea salt to a large saucepan. Heat the mixture until it's just bubbling and then remove from the heat and stir in the pecans. Pour the pecan mix over the baked shortbread crust and spread evenly.

5 Bake the bars for 10 minutes or until they start to bubble again. Remove from the oven and then cool for about 5 minutes. Sprinkle the dark chocolate chips over the top and then cool completely before slicing. Store at room temperature for four to five days or in the fridge for up to ten days. Wrap the bars well to store.

PER SERVING: *Calories 395; Fat 40g; Cholesterol 0mg; Sodium 68mg; Carbohydrates 28g (Dietary Fiber 8g, Sugar Alcohol 16g); Net Carbohydrates 4g; Protein 5g.*

BAKING KETO BROWNIES

Brownies are a genuine American concoction, which means they're perfect for Thanksgiving. They also make an excellent alternative for any chocolate lovers who may not be interested in a Thanksgiving pie. Choose dark, unsweetened chocolate to make your brownies fit your macros. You can also make fantastic brownies using just unsweetened cocoa powder and a keto sweetener of your choice. You really don't even need solid chocolate to make delicious brownies. Top your brownies with your choice of nuts or spread a chocolate frosting over the top. You can even make a keto ice cream recipe and serve it over the top of the brownies. Thanksgiving doesn't have to mean pie, and making deluxe brownies is a great alternative.

Chapter **16**

Crafting Keto Easter Treats

When Easter rolls around, it means spring is in the air. Most Easter desserts are light and delicious, reflecting the beautiful weather and brightness of the season. Spring is also an excellent time to focus on your keto diet because summer (and bathing suit season) is just around the corner. That doesn't mean that you have to abstain from desserts at Easter, though. The recipes in this chapter can help you have a great holiday in true, low-carb fashion.

Discovering Berries at Easter Time

As the weather warms, lots of awesome keto-friendly fruits start coming into season. Some of the following recipes utilize these fresh, springtime flavors to make your Easter treats festive and vibrant. Here are a few berries to consider:

» **Blueberries:** Blueberries are native to North America and Europe and are in season in the spring and summer, depending on where you live. They contain powerful antioxidants and are low in calories and carbs. Some of blueberries' powers include regulating blood sugar levels, helping improve memory, and enhancing overall brain health.

» **Raspberries:** Raspberries are part of the rose family with edible berries coming in red, black, and even golden varieties. Most raspberries grown in the United States are sourced from California, but they're actually native to Europe and Northern Asia. One cup of fresh raspberries has only 14 grams of carbs, which is much lower than many other fruits.

» **Strawberries:** Strawberries are one of the first fruits to appear in the springtime, showing their bright red color as soon as the weather begins to warm. These delicious treats are low in carbs and contain lots of vitamins and minerals, such as vitamin C, manganese, and folate. Strawberries bake wonderfully and are also perfect for making keto jams and jellies.

🍋 Lemon Raspberry Cheesecake

PREP TIME: 15 MIN | COOK TIME: 70–90 MIN | YIELD: 12 SERVINGS

INGREDIENTS

1 cup almond flour, finely ground

¼ cup butter, melted

2 tablespoons granular erythritol

½ cup coconut flour

1½ cups cream cheese, room temperature

¼ cup butter, room temperature

1 cup powdered erythritol

3 eggs, room temperature

¾ cup sour cream

½ tablespoon lemon extract

1 teaspoon lemon zest

1 cup fresh raspberries

DIRECTIONS

1 Preheat your oven to 300 degrees F. Grease a 9-inch, spring-form cake pan and place a round piece of parchment in the bottom of the pan. Wrap the outside of the pan with aluminum foil and then set the pan aside.

2 In a medium bowl, combine the almond flour, ¼ cup melted butter, 2 tablespoons granular erythritol, and coconut flour. Mix well and then pour into the prepared cake pan and press firmly into the bottom. Set aside.

3 Beat the cream cheese and ¼ cup butter together until light and fluffy. Add the powdered erythritol to the bowl and beat to combine well. Add the eggs one at a time, scraping down the sides of the bowl after each egg. Add the sour cream, lemon extract, and lemon zest and stir until a smooth batter forms. Fold in the fresh raspberries gently so as not to smash.

4 Pour the batter into the prepared pan and then place the pan in a water bath. Bake in the preheated oven for about 90 minutes. After 70 minutes, start checking to see whether the cheesecake has already set.

5 Remove the cheesecake from the oven and run a spatula around the edge of the pan to prevent the cake from sticking. Let the cheesecake cool completely before removing from the pan. Chill in the fridge before slicing and serving. Store the cheesecake in the fridge, wrapped well, for up to one week.

PER SERVING: *Calories 229; Fat 20g; Cholesterol 91mg; Sodium 71mg; Carbohydrates 25g (Dietary Fiber 3g, Sugar Alcohol 18g); Net Carbohydrates 3.3g; Protein 5.5g.*

NOTE: You'll know the cheesecake is set when the center jiggles slightly but is firm around the edges.

NOTE: If you're using frozen raspberries, mix them in while still frozen so that they don't turn the cheesecake pink.

Easter Egg Truffles

PREP TIME: 10 MIN	COOK TIME: 6 MIN	YIELD: 20 TRUFFLES

INGREDIENTS

1 cup sugar-free dark chocolate chips

¾ cup heavy whipping cream

3 tablespoons butter

4 tablespoons powdered erythritol

2 teaspoons maple extract

¼ cup unsweetened cocoa powder

DIRECTIONS

1 Place the chocolate chips in a large bowl and set aside. Add the heavy whipping cream, butter, and powdered erythritol to a small saucepan and heat over medium heat. Bring to a boil and then immediately remove from the heat. Pour the heavy whipping cream over the chocolate and let sit for 2 minutes. Whisk until smooth. Add the maple extract and stir.

2 Cover the bowl and let the chocolate cool to room temperature. It should be firm enough to scoop. Scoop into tablespoon-sized truffles, roll, and then use your hands to shape into an egg. Dip the egg in the cocoa powder and place on a tray.

3 Enjoy or store in an airtight container in the fridge for up to a week.

PER SERVING: *Calories 79; Fat 8g; Cholesterol 17mg; Sodium 4mg; Carbohydrates 8g (Dietary Fiber 3g, Sugar Alcohol 4g); Net Carbohydrates 1.7g; Protein 1g.*

EASTER EGGS ARE PERFECT KETO FOOD

Eggs happen to be a fantastic, keto-friendly food, and dying eggs is a longstanding Easter tradition. Eggs represent rebirth, which is a perfect reflection of the Easter holiday and the spring season when many plants and animals are "born again" as the weather warms. Eggs are dyed in a variety of colors, reflecting the brightness of spring. For many years, people would bring brightly decorated eggs to their family and friends as gifts at Easter. Save some eggs after you bake your Easter desserts and have fun dying (and then eating) them.

Carrot Cake Cupcakes

PREP TIME: 25 MIN	COOK TIME: 20 MIN	YIELD: 16 CUPCAKES

INGREDIENTS

¾ cup granular erythritol

¾ cup butter, softened

1 teaspoon vanilla extract

½ teaspoon pineapple extract (optional)

4 eggs, room temperature

2½ cups almond flour

2 teaspoons ground cinnamon

¾ teaspoon sea salt

2 teaspoons baking powder

2½ cups grated carrots

1½ cups chopped, toasted pecans

½ pound cream cheese, softened

¼ cup butter, softened

1 cup powdered erythritol

1 teaspoon vanilla extract

2 tablespoons heavy whipping cream

DIRECTIONS

1 Preheat your oven to 300 degrees F and place a cupcake liner in each cavity of a cupcake pan.

2 In a large bowl, blend the granular erythritol and butter until light and fluffy. Add the vanilla extract, pineapple extract, and the eggs, blending until fully combined. Add the almond flour, cinnamon, sea salt, and baking powder to the mix and blend well. Fold in the grated carrots and one cup of the pecans.

3 Scoop the batter into the prepared cupcake pan, filling each paper liner about ¾ of the way full. Bake the cupcakes for 20 minutes or until the cake springs back when pressed. Let cool in the tray completely and then move to a plate.

4 To make the frosting, beat the cream cheese, butter, and powdered erythritol together until smooth and fluffy. Add the vanilla extract and heavy whipping cream to the frosting and stir well.

5 Pipe the frosting over the top of each cupcake and then sprinkle with the remaining chopped pecans. Serve at room temperature or store in the fridge for up to five days.

PER SERVING: *Calories 399; Fat 9g; Cholesterol 102mg; Sodium 238mg; Carbohydrates 29g (Dietary Fiber 4g, Sugar Alcohol 21g); Net Carbohydrates 4.2g; Protein 8g.*

✆ Sugar-Free Gelatin Fluff

PREP TIME: 5 MIN | COOK TIME: 5 MIN | YIELD: 4 SERVINGS

INGREDIENTS

1 pack of sugar-free strawberry gelatin

1 cup water, boiling

4 ounces cream cheese, softened

2 cups crushed ice

½ cup heavy whipping cream

1 tablespoon powdered erythritol

DIRECTIONS

1 Place the gelatin powder in a medium bowl and add the boiling water. Stir until the gelatin has dissolved. Add the crushed ice and stir. The ice will melt, causing the gelatin to thicken. Once thick, remove any pieces of ice.

2 Beat the cream cheese in a large mixing bowl until smooth. Add the gelatin to the mixer, adding about ¼ cup at a time, beating after each addition. After all the gelatin has been added, the mix should be nice and fluffy. Scoop into serving dishes and let set in the fridge for at least 20 minutes before serving. If you plan to serve these fluffs later, keep them in the fridge (for up to three to four days) and top with the whipped cream right before serving.

3 Whip the heavy whipping cream and powdered erythritol until stiff peaks form. Scoop on top of each gelatin serving and enjoy.

PER SERVING: *Calories 204; Fat 21g; Cholesterol 72mg; Sodium 166mg; Carbohydrates 5g (Dietary Fiber 0g, Sugar Alcohol 3g); Net Carbohydrates 2g; Protein 3g.*

Adding Coconut to Your Easter Desserts

Coconut tends to find its way into a lot of springtime desserts. There is no specific reason as to why shredded coconut or coconut flavor in general is an Easter tradition, but it's definitely one we embrace because unsweetened coconut is perfect for a keto diet.

When choosing the coconut for these recipes, be sure to look for unsweetened coconut. The sweetened version has lots of added sugars (and therefore, carbs) that you want to avoid. But don't worry; coconut has its own natural sweetness that is present in any dessert you make that uses this ingredient. Coconut also adds some great, beneficial fats to each recipe that you want and need when on a keto diet, so have a nice big serving and enjoy these coconut Easter treats.

Tropical Carrot Cake

PREP TIME: 25 MIN	COOK TIME: 30 MIN	YIELD: 16 SERVINGS

INGREDIENTS

¾ cup granular erythritol

¾ cup coconut oil, softened

1 teaspoon coconut extract

4 eggs, room temperature

1½ cups almond flour

1 cup coconut flour

2 teaspoons ground cinnamon

¾ teaspoon sea salt

2 teaspoons baking powder

1½ cups grated carrots

1 cup unsweetened, shredded coconut flakes

1½ cups chopped, toasted walnuts

½ pound cream cheese, softened

¼ cup butter, softened

1 cup powdered erythritol

1 teaspoon coconut extract

2 tablespoons heavy whipping cream

DIRECTIONS

1 Preheat your oven to 300 degrees F and grease two 9-inch round pans, placing a piece of parchment paper in the bottom.

2 In a large bowl, blend the granular erythritol and coconut oil until light and fluffy. Add the coconut extract and the eggs, blending until fully combined. Add the almond flour, coconut flour, cinnamon, sea salt, and baking powder to the mix and blend well. Fold in the grated carrots, coconut flakes, and one cup of the walnuts.

3 Divide the batter between the two prepared pans and then bake in the preheated oven for 30 minutes or until completely set in the center. Allow the cakes to cool completely in the pans and then remove them and chill in the fridge for at least an hour.

4 To make the frosting, beat the cream cheese, butter, and powdered erythritol together until smooth and fluffy. Add the coconut extract and heavy whipping cream to the frosting and stir well. Spread a layer of frosting across the top of one of the carrot cakes and then place the second cake on top, sandwiching the frosting.

5 Frost the top of the cake and then sprinkle the remaining toasted walnuts. Slice and serve. Store the cake at room temperature for four to five days or in the fridge for up to one week.

PER SERVING: *Calories 299; Fat 28g; Cholesterol 79mg; Sodium 243mg; Carbohydrates 29g (Dietary Fiber 4g, Sugar Alcohol 21g); Net Carbohydrates 4g; Protein 5g.*

Coconut Cupcakes

PREP TIME: 10 MIN   COOK TIME: 25 MIN   YIELD: 10 SERVINGS

INGREDIENTS

5 eggs, room temperature, separated

¼ cup coconut flour

¼ cup almond flour

½ teaspoon sea salt

½ teaspoon xanthan gum

¼ cup granular erythritol

¼ cup butter, melted

¼ cup coconut oil, melted

1 teaspoon vanilla extract

8 ounces cream cheese, softened

¼ cup powdered erythritol

1 teaspoon vanilla extract

½ cup toasted shredded coconut, unsweetened

DIRECTIONS

1 Preheat your oven to 350 degrees F. Prepare a cupcake pan by placing a paper liner in each cupcake tin cavity and set aside.

2 Place the egg whites in a bowl and whip until stiff peaks form. Set aside. Add the coconut flour, almond flour, sea salt, xanthan gum and erythritol to a separate bowl and whisk together. Add the egg yolks, melted butter, melted coconut oil, and vanilla extract to the flour mix and stir together until a smooth batter forms. Fold the whipped egg whites into the batter gently and then scoop the batter into the cupcake pan, filling each cup about ¾ of the way full.

3 Bake for 25 minutes or until the cupcakes spring back to the touch. While the cake is baking, make the frosting by whipping the cream cheese and powdered erythritol together until light and fluffy. Add the vanilla extract and stir to combine.

4 After the cupcakes have cooled, remove from the pan and place on a tray. Scoop about 2 tablespoons frosting onto each cupcake. Dip the top of each cupcake in the toasted coconut, covering the frosting completely.

5 Serve the cupcakes at room temperature, storing wrapped for three to four days.

PER SERVING: *Calories 260; Fat 25g; Cholesterol 143mg; Sodium 245mg; Carbohydrates 14g (Dietary Fiber 2g, Sugar Alcohol 10g); Net Carbohydrates 2.6g; Protein 6g.*

Coconut Mousse Cups

PREP TIME: 5 MIN	COOK TIME: 8 MIN	YIELD: 6 SERVINGS

INGREDIENTS

1½ cups canned coconut cream

¼ cup granular erythritol

1 teaspoon vanilla extract

1 teaspoon coconut extract

1½ tablespoons gelatin powder

1½ cups heavy whipping cream

1 tablespoon unsweetened, shredded coconut, toasted

DIRECTIONS

1 Place the coconut cream, granular erythritol, vanilla extract, and coconut extract in a small saucepan and heat, stirring frequently, over medium heat. Once simmering, remove from the heat, stir in the gelatin to melt and cool to room temperature.

2 In a large mixing bowl, whip the heavy whipping cream until it forms stiff peaks. Add a scoop of the gelatin mix and continue to whisk. Keep adding the gelatin mix, whipping constantly, until all has been added.

3 Divide between serving cups, top with the shredded, toasted coconut and serve chilled.

PER SERVING: *Calories 152; Fat 15g; Cholesterol 27mg; Sodium 13mg; Carbohydrates 10g (Dietary Fiber 1g, Sugar Alcohol 8g); Net Carbohydrates 1.7g; Protein 3g.*

Chapter **17**

Commemorating December Holidays the Keto Way

D ecember should be considered the national month of baking. No matter what holiday you celebrate, more than likely you spend some days in December creating and sharing treats with family and friends. Whether you just started keto or have been a low-carb advocate for years, December can be a tough month. Carbohydrates seem to haunt you at every turn as sugar tries to push your name from the nice list to the naughty one. Don't worry. These recipes in this chapter allow you to enjoy all your favorite December desserts while staying on track with your low-carb macros.

Remembering Holiday Baking Traditions

Even though every family has its own holiday baking traditions, quite a few traditional desserts are common at this time of year. Here are a few that you may be interested in trying:

>> **Lebkuchen:** Lebkuchen is a traditional German spiced bar cookie. Filled with ginger, lemon, and orange flavors, it's a blast of holiday sensations. The bar is traditionally made by cooking brown sugar into a caramel and then mixing it into dry ingredients. Try using golden erythritol and almond flour for a keto-friendly version.

>> **Yule log:** This tradition began in Norway when a large log was placed on a fire to celebrate the year. Each family member would write a wish on a piece of paper, put it on the log, and then burn it. This tradition has been captured by baking a rolled cake (like the Gingerbread Roll Cake recipe in this chapter) and then decorating it to look like a log.

>> **Gingerbread:** Gingerbread houses began in Germany around the 16th century. Legend has it that Queen Elizabeth I came up with the idea to bake this delicious treat into houses and cookies, using gold leaf to make them elaborate and festive. This creation firmly cemented the taste of ginger as a holiday tradition.

>> **Mint desserts:** Candy canes became popular circa 1920 when a candy maker named Bob McCormack started turning straight candy sticks into a crook. His goal was to create a treat that reminded everyone of Jesus (hence the "J" shape when held one way and a shepherd's staff when held in reverse). The mint flavor is said to be symbolic of the hyssop plant that was used for purification in ancient times. Although these meanings were all applied after candy canes became popular, they've become part of Christmas lore. You can find many keto-friendly, sugar-free versions of this holiday treat.

Try the following keto classic December holiday recipes for your festivities.

🍅 Gingerbread Roll Cake

PREP TIME: 45 MIN	COOK TIME: 12 MIN	YIELD: 12 SERVINGS

INGREDIENTS

1 tablespoon gelatin

4 tablespoons water

1 cup finely ground almond flour

¼ cup powdered erythritol

2 tablespoons cocoa powder, unsweetened

¼ teaspoon ground cloves

2 teaspoons ground ginger

1 teaspoon ground cinnamon

4 eggs, separated

¼ cup granular erythritol

1 teaspoon vanilla extract

¼ teaspoon cream of tartar

¼ cup cream cheese, softened

1½ cups heavy whipping cream

¼ cup powdered erythritol

½ teaspoon vanilla extract

DIRECTIONS

1 Preheat oven to 350 degrees F. Line a rimmed 11x17 sheet tray with parchment paper.

2 Place the gelatin in a bowl with 4 tablespoons cold water and set aside to bloom. Whisk the almond flour, ¼ cup powdered erythritol, cocoa powder, cloves, ginger, and cinnamon together in a large mixing bowl. In a separate bowl, whip the egg yolks with 2 tablespoons granular erythritol until thick and light. Whisk in the vanilla extract and bloomed gelatin and set aside. In another bowl, whip the egg whites and cream of tartar until stiff peaks form. Fold the egg yolk mix into the egg whites and then gently fold in the dry ingredient mix. After the mix is blended, pour the batter into the prepared pan and spread flat and even.

3 Bake the cake in the preheated oven and cook for 10 to 12 minutes or until the top is set. While the cake is baking, make the frosting so you can frost it while still warm, making it easier to roll. Remove the cake from the oven and let cool completely. Remove the cake from the pan and place on your counter, keeping it in one large, flat piece.

4 Make the filling while the cake is baking by beating the cream cheese together with ¼ cup of the heavy whipping cream. In a separate bowl, whip the remaining heavy whipping cream, powdered erythritol, and vanilla extract until stiff peaks form. Fold the cream cheese and whipped cream together. Spread half of the filling over the top of the cake and then roll lengthwise into a tight log so the ends look like a spiral. Spread the remaining frosting on the outside of the roll, slice, and serve. Wrap the cake well and store at room temperature for three to four days or in the fridge for up to one week.

PER SERVING: *Calories 137; Fat 12g; Cholesterol 90mg; Sodium 47mg; Carbohydrates 15g (Dietary Fiber 1g, Sugar Alcohol 12g); Net Carbohydrates 1.9g; Protein 5g.*

Eggnog Cheesecake Fat Bombs

PREP TIME: 20 MIN	COOK TIME: 30 MIN	YIELD: 12 FAT BOMBS

INGREDIENTS

½ cup finely ground almond flour

¼ cup ground flaxseeds

2 tablespoons powdered erythritol

¼ teaspoon ground nutmeg

2 tablespoons butter, melted

1 egg

¾ pound cream cheese, softened

½ cup powdered erythritol

1 tablespoon rum extract

½ teaspoon vanilla extract

1 egg

½ cup heavy whipping cream

¼ teaspoon ground nutmeg

DIRECTIONS

1 Preheat your oven to 325 degrees F and prepare a cupcake tray with paper cupcake liners.

2 In a large bowl, combine the almond flour, flaxseeds, powdered erythritol, and nutmeg. Add the melted butter and the egg to the almond flour mix and stir until crumbly.

3 Scoop the mixture into the prepared cupcake liners and then press down, firmly compacting the crust. Bake in the oven for 10 minutes to brown lightly. Remove and let the crusts cool.

4 Put the cream cheese, ½ cup powdered erythritol, rum extract, and vanilla extract in a bowl and beat until smooth. Add the egg, heavy whipping cream, and nutmeg and blend again.

5 Pour the cream cheese mixture into the cupcake liners, dividing the batter evenly between the prepared crusts. Bake for 16 to 18 minutes or until the centers are set. Remove from the oven and cool for at least 1 hour in the fridge. Store wrapped in the fridge for up to one week.

PER SERVING: *Calories 202; Fat 19g; Cholesterol 85mg; Sodium 119mg; Carbohydrates 13g (Dietary Fiber 1g, Sugar Alcohol 10g); Net Carbohydrates 2g; Protein 5g.*

Low-Carb Fruitcake

PREP TIME: 15 MIN	COOK TIME: 30 MIN	YIELD: 14 SERVINGS

INGREDIENTS

4 eggs, room temperature

¼ cup butter, melted

1 tablespoon vanilla extract

⅓ cup granular erythritol

1 tablespoon orange zest

1½ cups finely ground almond flour

½ teaspoon baking soda

½ cup dried cranberries

1 cup chopped walnuts

DIRECTIONS

1 Preheat your oven to 350 degrees F and line a loaf pan with parchment strips in the bottom. Whisk together the eggs, melted butter, vanilla extract, granular erythritol, and orange zest. Add the almond flour and baking soda, whisking until smooth. Fold in the cranberries and walnuts until well mixed and then pour the batter into the prepared loaf pan.

2 Bake for about 30 minutes or until a toothpick comes out cleanly when inserted in the center of the cake. Remove the pan from the oven and cool in the pan for about 30 minutes and then remove the cake from the pan and cool completely on a wire rack. Slice and serve. Store in the fridge for up to one week.

PER SERVING: *Calories 192; Fat 16g; Cholesterol 69mg; Sodium 111mg; Carbohydrates 12g (Dietary Fiber 2g, Sugar Alcohol 4g); Net Carbohydrates 5.2g; Protein 6g.*

Chocolate Peppermint Shortbread

PREP TIME: 30 MIN | COOK TIME: 30 MIN | YIELD: 12 SERVINGS

INGREDIENTS

¼ cup butter, softened

⅓ cup granular erythritol

½ teaspoon vanilla extract

1⅔ cups finely ground almond flour

1 tablespoon coconut oil

1 cup dark chocolate chips, unsweetened

2 teaspoons peppermint extract

3 tablespoons crushed sugar-free peppermint candies (optional)

DIRECTIONS

1 Preheat your oven to 350 degrees F and line a small 6x8-inch casserole dish with parchment paper.

2 Beat the butter and granular erythritol together in a bowl until light and fluffy. Add the vanilla extract and beat to combine. Mix in the almond flour until a thick dough forms.

3 Press the dough into the prepared pan and then bake until the shortbread begins to turn golden brown, about 25 minutes. Remove the shortbread from the oven and let cool completely.

4 Place the coconut oil, dark chocolate chips, and peppermint extract in a bowl and melt over a double boiler, stirring frequently until smooth. Spread the melted chocolate over the top of the cooled shortbread and then sprinkle with the crushed peppermints (if using). After the chocolate has set, slice and serve. Store in an airtight container at room temperature for up to one week.

PER SERVING: *Calories 133; Fat 13g; Cholesterol 10mg; Sodium 1mg; Carbohydrates 16g (Dietary Fiber 5g, Sugar Alcohol 9g); Net Carbohydrates 2.6g; Protein 2g.*

🍅 Hazelnut Truffles

PREP TIME: 20 MIN	COOK TIME: 5 MIN	YIELD: 16 SERVINGS

INGREDIENTS

¼ cup toasted hazelnuts

1 teaspoon powdered erythritol

2 teaspoons coconut oil, melted

1 teaspoon unsweetened cocoa powder

1 teaspoon water (if needed)

⅓ cup coconut oil

½ cup dark chocolate chips, unsweetened

⅓ cup powdered erythritol

½ teaspoon vanilla extract

½ cup finely chopped, toasted hazelnuts

DIRECTIONS

1 Place the hazelnuts, 1 teaspoon powdered erythritol, 2 teaspoons coconut oil, and 1 teaspoon cocoa powder in a food processor and pulse until smooth. Place the hazelnut blend, coconut oil, dark chocolate chips, ⅓ cup powdered erythritol, and vanilla extract in a small saucepan.

2 Heat over medium low heat, stirring constantly until smooth and completely melted. Pour the mix into a bowl and place in the fridge for about an hour or until completely set.

3 After set, scoop the truffles into tablespoon-sized balls and roll with your hands to make round. Roll each truffle in the chopped hazelnuts to coat the outside.

4 Store in the refrigerator for up to one week until you're ready to enjoy.

PER SERVING: *Calories 99; Fat 10g; Cholesterol 0mg; Sodium 0mg; Carbohydrates 9g (Dietary Fiber 2g, Sugar Alcohol 5g); Net Carbohydrates 1.2g; Protein 1g.*

TIP: If needed, add a teaspoon of water after pulsing the hazelnuts, powdered erythritol, coconut oil, and cocoa powder to make the mix creamier. You want it to be the consistency of smooth peanut butter.

🍅 Cranberry Swirl Cheesecake

PREP TIME: 25 MIN   COOK TIME: 90 MIN   YIELD: 12 SERVINGS

INGREDIENTS

6 ounces fresh cranberries

½ cup powdered erythritol

⅓ cup water

½ teaspoon orange zest

½ teaspoon vanilla extract

1½ cups cream cheese, room temperature

¼ cup butter, room temperature

1 cup powdered erythritol

3 eggs, room temperature

¾ cup sour cream

½ teaspoon vanilla extract

DIRECTIONS

1   Place the cranberries, ½ cup powdered erythritol, water, orange zest, and ½ teaspoon vanilla extract in a small saucepan and bring to a boil over medium heat. Simmer for about 10 minutes to thicken. Set the cranberry sauce aside to cool completely.

2   Preheat your oven to 300 degrees F. Grease a 7-inch, spring-form cake pan and place a round piece of parchment in the bottom of the pan. Wrap the outside of the pan with aluminum foil and then set the pan aside.

3   Beat the cream cheese and butter together until light and fluffy. Add 1 cup powdered erythritol to the bowl and beat to combine well. Add the eggs one at a time, scraping down the sides of the bowl after each addition. Add the sour cream and vanilla extract and stir until a smooth batter forms. Pour the batter into the prepared pan and then place the pan in a water bath.

4   Scoop the cranberry sauce into the cheesecake pan, placing the scoops apart from each other so cranberry is in every section of the cake.

5   Bake in the preheated oven for about 90 minutes. After 70 minutes, start checking to see if the cheesecake has already set.

6   Remove the cheesecake from the oven and run a spatula around the edge of the pan to prevent the cake from sticking. Let the cheesecake cool completely before removing from the pan. Chill in the fridge before slicing and serving. Store in the refrigerator for up to one week.

PER SERVING: *Calories 187; Fat 18g; Cholesterol 103mg; Sodium 131mg; Carbohydrates 27g (Dietary Fiber 1g, Sugar Alcohol 24g); Net Carbohydrates 2.8g; Protein 4g.*

NOTE: In Step 4, use a knife to gently swirl the cranberry sauce into the cheesecake, being careful to just swirl and not completely mix it in.

NOTE: The cheesecake is set when the center slightly jiggles but is firm around the edges.

Chocolate Pots de Crème

| PREP TIME: 15 MIN | COOK TIME: 10 MIN | YIELD: 4 SERVINGS |

INGREDIENTS

4 ounces dark baking chocolate

1 cup canned coconut milk, full fat

¾ cup powdered erythritol

2 egg yolks, room temperature

1 teaspoon vanilla extract

DIRECTIONS

1 Chop the dark chocolate and place in a small saucepan. Add the coconut milk and powdered erythritol in the saucepan and bring to a simmer over low heat. Whisk to combine and make the mixture smooth.

2 In a separate bowl, whisk together the eggs and vanilla extract. Slowly add in the melted chocolate mixture into the eggs, whisking constantly. Pour the chocolate and egg mix back into the saucepan and heat over low for 1 more minute, whisking constantly.

3 Pour the chocolate mix into four small dishes or ramekins and then place in the fridge to chill for at least three hours. Enjoy chilled.

PER SERVING: *Calories 157; Fat 14g; Cholesterol 92mg; Sodium 7mg; Carbohydrates 55g (Dietary Fiber 8g, Sugar Alcohol 42g); Net Carbohydrates 5g; Protein 4g.*

Loving Christmas Cookies

Above all other desserts, the idea of cookies during the holiday season is by far the most popular. Although accounts vary as to why cookies are popular, the most common story traces their roots to children leaving cookies and milk for St. Nick on Christmas Eve. Tradition holds that children placed snacks out to fuel Santa Claus on his journey as well as thank him for the presents he left. Of course, there are many other reasons why cookies are a Christmas tradition, and you don't need to skip out because many keto cookies are available. We have some great keto cookie recipes you can enjoy. You can also use our recipes in this section to make some of these Christmas classics.

⏲ Low-Carb Praline Cookies

| PREP TIME: 15 MIN | COOK TIME: 0 MIN | YIELD: ABOUT 20 COOKIES |

INGREDIENTS

½ cup heavy whipping cream

4 tablespoons butter, softened

½ cup granular erythritol

1 tablespoon coconut oil

1 teaspoon vanilla extract

1 cup unsweetened, shredded coconut

1 cup chopped pecans, toasted

DIRECTIONS

1 Add the heavy whipping cream, butter, granular erythritol, and coconut oil to a large saucepan and bring to a boil over medium heat. Lower the heat and let the mix simmer for 10 minutes. The mix should be a light golden brown. Remove the pan from the heat and add the vanilla extract, coconut, and pecans and stir well.

2 Scoop the mixture into tablespoon-sized scoops, placing on a parchment-lined sheet tray. Set the pralines in the freezer until firm, about 30 minutes. Store in an airtight container in the freezer for up to a month or fridge for up to two weeks.

PER SERVING: *Calories 129; Fat 13g; Cholesterol 14mg; Sodium 4mg; Carbohydrates 7g (Dietary Fiber 2g, Sugar Alcohol 5g); Net Carbohydrates .4g; Protein 1g.*

TIP: Dip the cookies into melted, unsweetened chocolate and then place on a lined sheet tray to dry. Enjoy the extra chocolate taste and decadence.

Chocolate Rugelach

INGREDIENTS

1 cup finely ground almond flour

¼ cup coconut flour

½ teaspoon xanthan gum

½ cup butter

¼ cup cream cheese, softened

1 egg

1 teaspoon vanilla extract

2 tablespoons apple cider vinegar

1 cup unsweetened dark chocolate chips

2 tablespoons unsweetened cocoa powder

2 tablespoons granular erythritol

1 teaspoon butter

DIRECTIONS

1 Preheat your oven to 350 degrees F.

2 Pulse to combine the almond flour, coconut flour, and xanthan gum in a food processor. Add the butter and cream cheese to the food processor and pulse until the mixture is crumbly. Add the egg, vanilla extract, and apple cider vinegar and pulse until the mix looks like breadcrumbs. Divide the dough into two separate balls, wrap tightly, and refrigerate for at least an hour to chill.

3 After chilled, roll each ball of dough separately between two pieces of parchment paper, keeping the dough rectangular as you roll. Place the two rectangles in the fridge while you make the filling.

4 Place the dark chocolate chips, cocoa powder, granular erythritol, and butter in a small microwavable bowl. Microwave for 30 seconds, stir, and repeat, microwaving in 30-second increments until melted and smooth. Let cool slightly.

5 Remove one of the dough rectangles from the fridge and spread half of the chocolate mixture across the entire dough. Roll the dough into a long log and then wrap in the parchment again and place back in the fridge. Repeat with the other dough rectangle and filling.

6 After the logs have chilled, remove them from the fridge and slice into ½-inch thick pieces, placing them on a parchment-lined sheet tray to bake.

7 Bake for 15 minutes or until the edges of the cookies are beginning to brown. Remove from the oven and cool completely. Store in an airtight container in the fridge for up to two weeks.

PER SERVING: *Calories 209; Fat 19g; Cholesterol 43mg; Sodium 32mg; Carbohydrates 14g (Dietary Fiber 6g, Sugar Alcohol 4g); Net Carbohydrates 3.8g; Protein 5g.*

VARY IT: Use keto raspberry jam inside the rugelach dough rather than the chocolate filling.

Chapter **18**

Bringing In New Year's with a Keto Bang

t's the end of the year, and you need to celebrate. What better way to kick off the new year than with a delicious, flavorful, keto-friendly dessert? January 1 is the most popular day of the year to begin a new diet. Although many people don't make their resolutions last, your chances are much better because you have this book. One of the most common reasons diet resolutions fail is a lack of preparation and support, both of which we address in this book and chapter. This chapter gives you many options that are perfect for a New Year's Eve party, a small get-together, or even a night alone. No matter how you spend the new year, make sure your taste buds are included in the party.

Gathering with Keto Desserts

Many of these recipes in this section are perfect for a party or gathering, something many people attend on New Year's. The Champagne cupcakes, for example, are sure to be a party hit and no one will even notice that they are missing the usual amount of carbs — they just taste so good! So raise a glass and raise a keto dessert as well to a positive, healthy new beginning.

⌣ Champagne Cupcakes

PREP TIME: 30 MIN	COOK TIME: 25 MIN	YIELD: 12 SERVINGS

INGREDIENTS

2 cups finely ground, blanched almond flour

½ cup coconut flour

¼ teaspoon sea salt

1 teaspoon baking soda

1 teaspoon baking powder

4 eggs, room temperature

⅔ cup granular erythritol

⅔ cup butter, melted and cooled

1½ teaspoons lemon extract

½ teaspoon vanilla extract

1 tablespoon lemon zest

¼ cup dry champagne

½ cup unsweetened coconut milk, canned

½ pound cream cheese, softened

½ cup softened butter

⅔ cup powdered erythritol

½ cup dry champagne

DIRECTIONS

1 Preheat your oven to 350 degrees F and prepare a cupcake tray with paper cupcake liners.

2 Combine the almond flour, coconut flour, sea salt, baking soda, and baking powder in a large bowl, whisk together, and then set aside. In a separate bowl, combine the eggs, granular erythritol, melted butter, both extracts, lemon zest, and the dry champagne and whisk together well. Add the coconut milk to the wet ingredients and whisk again. Add the dry ingredients to the wet mixture slowly, adding only about half a cup at a time and whisking well after each addition to ensure everything is well blended and no lumps form.

3 Scoop the batter into the cupcake tray, filling each paper liner about three-quarters of the way up the sides. Place in the preheated oven to bake for 30 minutes or until a toothpick comes out of the center of the cake cleanly and the tops of the cakes are a golden brown. Allow the cupcakes to cool completely.

4 Place the remaining ½ cup dry champagne in a small saucepan and bring to a boil. Cook for 5 minutes to reduce and thicken. Set aside to cool completely.

5 Place the cream cheese, butter, and powdered erythritol in a stand mixer and beat until light and fluffy. Add the cooled champagne and then blend together with the frosting, mixing until fully incorporated. Top each cupcake with the frosting, piping or spreading it on evenly. Store in an airtight container in the fridge for four to five days.

PER SERVING: *Calories 394; Fat 36g; Cholesterol 138mg; Sodium 283mg; Carbohydrates 19g (Dietary Fiber 4g, Sugar Alcohol 11g); Net Carbohydrates 4.1g; Protein 8g.*

⌒ Coconut Chocolate Bark

PREP TIME: 4 MIN	COOK TIME: 10 MIN	YIELD: 14 SERVINGS

INGREDIENTS

¾ cup sliced almonds

½ cup unsweetened shredded coconut

¾ pound dark baking chocolate

DIRECTIONS

1 Place the sliced almonds and coconut on a parchment-lined sheet tray and toast in the oven until golden (about 5 to 10 minutes in a 350 degrees F oven). Set aside to cool.

2 Melt the dark chocolate over a double boiler, stirring constantly until smooth. Spread the chocolate on a silicone mat on a flat sheet tray. Sprinkle the almonds and coconut over the top of the chocolate.

3 Place the tray in the fridge to set and then break into pieces. Store in an airtight container in the fridge for up to three weeks.

PER SERVING: *Calories 178; Fat 16g; Cholesterol 0mg; Sodium 3mg; Carbohydrates 19g (Dietary Fiber 10g, Sugar Alcohol 5g); Net Carbohydrates 3.9g; Protein 3g.*

☕ Espresso Rum Truffles

| PREP TIME: 10 MIN | COOK TIME: 6 MIN | YIELD: 20 TRUFFLES |

INGREDIENTS

1¼ cups sugar-free dark chocolate chips

¾ cup heavy whipping cream

3 tablespoons butter

5 tablespoons powdered erythritol

1 teaspoon rum extract

1 teaspoon coffee extract or 2 tablespoons brewed espresso

¼ cup unsweetened cocoa powder

DIRECTIONS

1 Place the chocolate in a large bowl and set aside. Add the heavy whipping cream, butter, and powdered erythritol to a small saucepan and heat over medium heat. Bring to a boil and then immediately remove from the heat. Pour the cream over the chocolate and let sit for 2 minutes. Whisk until smooth. Add the rum extract and coffee extract or brewed espresso and stir.

2 Cover the bowl and let the chocolate cool to room temperature. Scoop into tablespoon-sized truffles and roll into small balls with your hands. Dip the truffles in the cocoa powder and place on a tray.

3 Roll and shape all the truffles and then enjoy or store in an airtight container in the fridge for up to a week.

PER SERVING: *Calories 87; Fat 9g; Cholesterol 17mg; Sodium 4mg; Carbohydrates 11g (Dietary Fiber 3g, Sugar Alcohol 5g); Net Carbohydrates 2g; Protein 1g.*

NOTE: The chocolate mixture in Step 2 should cool long enough so it's firm to scoop.

Coconut Squares

INGREDIENTS

3 cups shredded unsweetened coconut

¼ cup liquid stevia

¼ cup melted coconut oil

⅓ cup melted butter

1 teaspoon vanilla extract

¼ teaspoon sea salt

DIRECTIONS

1 Line an 8x8-inch square pan with a piece of parchment.

2 Mix together the coconut, liquid stevia, melted coconut oil, melted butter, vanilla extract, and sea salt. Stir until thick. Press the mixture into the prepared pan, compacting it evenly in the pan.

3 Place in the fridge or freezer until completely cooled. Slice and enjoy. Store in the fridge in an airtight container for up to one month.

PER SERVING: *Calories 183; Fat 18g; Cholesterol 8mg; Sodium 32mg; Carbohydrates 5g (Dietary Fiber 5g, Sugar Alcohol 0g); Net Carbohydrates 0g; Protein 1.2g.*

Creating Some New Year's Eve Desserts

New Year's Eve is a time to celebrate all your accomplishments from the past year and also to look forward to the new and exciting adventures in the year to come. Such a big, celebratory day deserves amazing desserts, and we have plenty of them for you. If you're already following a keto diet or looking to start one in the new year, these desserts can also help you stick to those resolutions while still indulging in something delicious.

CHOOSING NEW YEAR'S EVE FOODS

Traditional New Year's Eve dishes are numerous and vary by culture. What they all have in common is that they're assumed to bring luck as you welcome the next 12 months. Many are keto-friendly, so don't hesitate to give some a try. Who knows? They may even bring you good fortune. Here are some of the more common ones:

- **Greens:** Greens are considered to be good luck when eaten on New Year's Eve. The green color resembles money, and financial motivation is one of the main reasons this tradition has carried on. Try collard greens, kale, or spinach, all of which are keto-approved.

- **Pork:** Pork is believed to be lucky to eat because pigs are round, indicating a fat wallet. They also have a unique eating style and are continually walking forward as they munch on goodies, which symbolizes continued progress. The cuts of meat are fattier, which is indicative of prosperity. The best news? Pork is perfect for any keto dieter.

- **Fish:** The scales on a fish resemble coins, which is why it's said to be lucky to eat fish on New Year's. Fish also swim in schools, representing abundance. Try a great fish recipe to usher in some good luck in the new year.

- **Oranges:** Oranges are the main symbol of the Chinese New Year and are believed to bring prosperity. Having a stem and leaf attached to the orange is supposed to usher in long life and fertility. A slice or two of this fresh fruit tastes great and hopefully brings you good luck. Oranges are high in carbs, but they're low enough that a slice or two won't hurt.

Crème Brulee

PREP TIME: 10 MIN	COOK TIME: 35 MIN	YIELD: 4 SERVINGS

INGREDIENTS

4 egg yolks

1 teaspoon vanilla extract

2 cups heavy whipping cream

1 tablespoon granular erythritol

2 tablespoons golden erythritol

DIRECTIONS

1 Preheat your oven to 325 degrees F.

2 Whisk the egg yolks and vanilla extract in a large mixing bowl and set aside. Place the heavy whipping cream and granular erythritol in a small saucepan and bring to a simmer over low heat. Slowly pour the hot cream into the bowl with the egg yolks, whisking constantly. Pour the mix into four ramekins and then place the ramekins in a water bath.

3 Bake in the oven for 30 minutes or until the center of the crème brulee is set. Let the crème brulee cool and then sprinkle the tops with the golden erythritol.

4 Use a culinary torch to heat the sweetener and caramelize each ramekin; stop when the erythritol begins to turn a light brown. Serve immediately.

PER SERVING: *Calories 468; Fat 49g; Cholesterol 348mg; Sodium 54mg; Carbohydrates 13g (Dietary Fiber 0g, Sugar Alcohol 9g); Net Carbohydrates 4.1g; Protein 5g.*

Raspberry Chocolate Cheesecake Bars

PREP TIME: 15 MIN	COOK TIME: 25 MIN	YIELD: 9 SERVINGS

INGREDIENTS

1 cup cream cheese, softened

½ cup powdered erythritol

1 egg

1 teaspoon vanilla extract

½ cup fresh raspberries

⅔ cup granular erythritol

¾ cup unsweetened cocoa powder

½ cup almond flour

¼ cup coconut flour

3 eggs

½ cup butter, melted

1 tablespoon vanilla extract

2 tablespoons unsweetened almond milk

DIRECTIONS

1 Preheat your oven to 350 degrees F and prepare an 8x8-inch cake pan with parchment paper.

2 Place the cream cheese, powdered erythritol, 1 egg, 1 teaspoon vanilla extract, and ½ cup raspberries in a food processor and pulse until smooth.

3 In a separate bowl, combine the ⅔ cup granular erythritol, cocoa powder, almond flour, and coconut flour and whisk together. Add the eggs, butter, 1 tablespoon vanilla extract, and almond milk and whisk until a smooth batter forms. Pour the chocolate batter into the prepared pan and then top with the raspberry cheesecake mix. Gently swirl together the chocolate and raspberry mix with a knife.

4 Bake for 25 minutes or until completely set in the center. Let the bars cool completely and then slice. Store in the fridge in an airtight container for up to two days.

PER SERVING: *Calories 287; Fat 26g; Cholesterol 150mg; Sodium137mg; Carbohydrates 34g (Dietary Fiber 5g, Sugar Alcohol 25g); Net Carbohydrates 4.5g; Protein 8g.*

🌰 Almond Semifreddo

PREP TIME: 50 MIN	COOK TIME: 10 MIN	YIELD: 10 SERVINGS

INGREDIENTS

1 cup raspberries

¼ cup granular erythritol

2 tablespoons lemon juice

⅛ teaspoon ground cinnamon

1 teaspoon almond extract

2 tablespoons water

4 cups heavy whipping cream

¼ cup powdered erythritol

2 teaspoons vanilla extract

½ teaspoon almond extract

3 tablespoons powdered erythritol

2 tablespoons vanilla vodka, no sugar added

1 teaspoon almond extract

4 egg yolks

4 egg whites

¼ cup powdered erythritol

⅛ teaspoon cream of tartar

DIRECTIONS

1 Place the raspberries, ¼ cup granular erythritol, lemon juice, cinnamon, 1 teaspoon almond extract, and water in a small saucepan. Bring to a boil and cook for about 10 minutes to thicken. Place in a blender and puree until smooth and then set aside to cool.

2 Place the heavy whipping cream and ¼ cup powdered erythritol into a bowl and whip until stiff peaks form. Add the vanilla extract and ½ teaspoon almond extract. Whip together and set aside. Place a bowl over a double boiler and add the 3 tablespoons powdered erythritol, vodka, and teaspoon almond extract. Stir to heat.

3 Place a bowl over a double boiler and add the 3 tablespoons powdered erythritol, vodka, and teaspoon almond extract. Stir to heat.

4 Add the egg yolks and whisk over the double boiler, heating and whipping the eggs at the same time to prevent them from cooking completely. Use a hand mixer to beat the eggs over the double boiler until thick and tripled in volume. Remove from the heat and pour into a new bowl to cool.

5 Place the egg whites, ¼ cup powdered erythritol, and cream of tartar over a double boiler as well (you can use the pot of water from the first double boil you used in Step 3). Whip until stiff while over the heat to cook and thicken. When the whites are thick and shiny, remove from the heat.

6 Line a loaf pan with plastic wrap.

(continued)

7 Stir the whipped cream mix and the egg yolk mix together gently. Then, fold the egg whites in gently. Spread about a third of the mix into the prepared pan. Spread half of the raspberry sauce over the whipped cream mix. Add another third of the whipped cream mix and then spread the remaining raspberry sauce in the pan. Add the remaining whipped mixture and then take a knife and swirl it together gently.

8 Place the pan in the freezer and chill until solid. When ready to serve, use the plastic wrap to lift the semifreddo out of the pan. Slice and serve. Store in the fridge for up to two days.

PER SERVING: *Calories 377; Fat 37g; Cholesterol 204mg; Sodium 62mg; Carbohydrates 23g (Dietary Fiber 1g, Sugar Alcohol 18g); Net Carbohydrates 4g; Protein 5g.*

4

The Part of Tens

Discover the best sweeteners for each dessert, exploring their various properties, and understanding the impact each has on your baking. Knowing how to work with new ingredients and combinations makes all the difference in creating low-carb dessert delicacies.

Experience a brief overview of numerous additional resources, from sites that focus on food prep with allergies or medical limitations to publications that can help you customize keto for kids. There's something in this list for everyone, so dig in and find the information that is the most beneficial for your unique situation.

Chapter **19**

Top Ten Most Common Keto Sweeteners

A keto dessert book would be lost without a discussion on artificial sweeteners. Not all sweeteners have the same properties, however, and understanding the ins and outs of each one is crucial to ensure you select the right option for you. Sweeteners vary in taste, consistency, baking behavior, and the effect they have on your digestive system. Although you won't need to have all ten of these on hand, you'll probably want to pick two or three that become your defaults.

Some artificial sweeteners have a reputation for causing upset stomachs, bloating, cramps, and diarrhea. The primary reason is the sheer amount of artificial sweeteners that a person would need to consume to trigger this effect. The average American consumes between 150 and 170 pounds of sugar per year; replacing that with something like erythritol is infinitely better, but consuming that amount of anything is going to upset your stomach. However, replacing your sugar intake with a quality sweetener while simultaneously decreasing your overall intake of sweet treats will minimize your chances of experiencing any GI issues.

Erythritol

Erythritol is a sugar alcohol that naturally occurs in pears, watermelon, soy sauce, and a variety of other fruits and vegetables, and it's one that we highly recommend. The kind that you buy in the store is typically synthesized from corn glucose. Although it starts as a sugar, the fermentation process changes the chemical composition of the alcohol. Your tongue will still taste that it's sweet, but your body won't recognize it as sugar.

One of the typical benefits of most sugar alcohols is that they don't break down in your digestive system, preventing your body from metabolizing them and creating a rise in blood sugar. Erythritol is typically passed into the gut and then excreted through urine in a virtually unprocessed state. This particular sugar alcohol tends to behave just like sugar. It can be used as replacement, and it creates similar effects to processed sugar in most recipes.

Monk Fruit Extract

Monk fruit extract comes straight from a small, round, green fruit that is almost exclusively located in China. It's an unusual plant because, unlike virtually all other fruits, its sweetness doesn't come from fructose. Instead, monk fruit is characterized by antioxidants called *mogrosides*. Monk fruit extract doesn't impact blood glucose levels at all, despite tasting 300 to 400 times sweeter than sugar.

One of the crucial aspects of monk fruit extract is knowing what form works best for how you're using it. It's generally sold in either a powder or liquid form, and because it's so sweet, a little goes a long way. This can make measurements a bit difficult, so this sweetener is often blended with sugar alcohols to create a granular substance that looks similar to regular white sugar and can be used as a 1:1 or 2:1 replacement. This sweetener should also be at the top of your list.

Stevia

Another plant-based sugar substitute, stevia is derived from the leaves of the stevia plant, found in Paraguay and Brazil. Its sweetness stems from *steviol glycosides,* which aren't metabolized by the body and therefore have no effect on blood glucose levels. Although much sweeter than sugar, it takes a bit longer to taste the sweetness, but that taste sticks around for longer than sugar would.

Although stevia can be readily purchased in granular form, you don't need nearly as much of it as you would sugar in a recipe. Hence, you may need to make some adjustments to compensate for the bulk of dry ingredients you're missing.

Xylitol

Xylitol is another sugar alcohol that is naturally found in plums, strawberries, pumpkin, and cauliflower. It's commonly synthesized from the by-products of corn, wheat, or rice in commercial production. It's absorbed by the body and has an impact on your blood glucose, although that impact is far less pronounced than the effect sugar has. Xylitol is relatively simple to use in baking. It's produced in such a way that it can be used as a 1:1 replacement for sugar so measurements are straightforward. It handles heat well, but it doesn't caramelize like regular sugar, which can impact some dessert recipes.

Truvia

Truvia is a combination of stevia and erythritol, creating a granular substance that appears virtually identical to sugar. In nonbaking applications, Truvia can be used by itself, but when it comes to baking, you need to use three-quarters Truvia and one-quarter actual sugar. If you don't, your baking won't turn out as you expect. Because of this, Truvia is a sweetener we recommend only for nonbaking uses.

Sucralose

Sucralose starts with sucrose, which is a combination of glucose and fructose. It's then chlorinated, eventually arriving at a chemical composition that is 300 times sweeter than sugar, but the body doesn't break it down. This sweetener begins to break down at temperatures higher than 250 degrees Fahrenheit, making it a poor choice for baking. It is, however, an excellent sugar substitute for low-temperature recipes.

Splenda

Splenda is a combination of sucralose, dextrose, and maltodextrin. The sweetness comes from the first, whereas the latter two are used as bulking agents to give Splenda a usable volume. Splenda tastes as sweet as sugar and contains one-third of the calories. It's allowed to be listed as a zero-calorie sweetener because the calories are so low, but in larger amounts, they can add up. This sugar alternative is excellent for baking and avoids the aftertaste that many artificial sweeteners have. It's stable at high temperatures, but it doesn't brown or caramelize the way regular sugar does, which can be either critical or irrelevant, depending on the effect you're trying to achieve.

Yacon Syrup

Yacon syrup is derived from the roots of the yacon plant, which is indigenous to the Andes Mountains. Its natural sweetness comes from *fructooligosaccharides*, which naturally don't impact blood sugar. The most distinguishing characteristic of this sweetener is its taste, which is similar to molasses or caramelized sugar, making this sweetener valuable for some specific dessert uses.

Aspartame

Aspartame is a chemical composition first discovered in 1965. Although it has a negative reputation, it's one of the most rigorously tested food ingredients and has been determined by the FDA to be safe for consumption at normal levels. It can create a rise in blood glucose, but that rise is so low that it's negligible. Aspartame does tend to break down at higher temperatures. We don't recommend it for baking, although you can add it to a recipe near the end of a baking cycle.

Saccharin

A chemical composition formally known as benzoic sulfimide, *saccharin* is most commonly combined with other artificial sweeteners. It doesn't impact blood glucose, is heat stable, and can be useful for baking, although it tends to create a bitter aftertaste in high concentrations. The most common uses of saccharin, beyond sweetener blends, are diet sodas and medicine.

Chapter **20**

Top Ten Resources for Keto Dessert Recipes

C ooking and baking are every bit as much of an art as they are a science, and part of having a vibrant food experience is regularly experiencing new recipes and cooking styles. This chapter lists ten of our favorite resources for keto desserts. Many of them have specific focuses, from vegan cooking to a dairy-free approach — there's something for everyone in this chapter.

Tasteaholics and So Nourished

We fell in love with keto and launched Tasteaholics (www.tasteaholics.com) to share our low-carb journey with the world. The driving purpose behind every piece of content we created was the question: "What would we have liked to have as a resource when we first started?" We've packed these sites with informational resources as well as hundreds of free recipes. Our passion is to help others enjoy the health benefits that have so revolutionized our own lives, and we want to give you everything you need to be able to do that.

So Nourished (www.sonourished.com) was a natural offshoot as we realized we couldn't find some of the keto products we were looking for — so we made our own! Many of these products were driven by the desire to create delicious low-carb desserts, so we created proprietary blends of keto sweeteners that make baking so much easier.

Low Carb Yum

Lisa MarcAurele has a passion for low-carb living. When she began her keto journey well over a decade ago, she wasn't much of a cook. She relied heavily on processed foods and canned ingredients as crutches, but soon discovered that making everything from scratch was half the fun! Her site (www.lowcarbyum.com) focuses not only on low-carb recipes but also ensures that every dish she creates is gluten-free. Many of her recipes are dairy-free, paleo (including the autoimmune protocol), nut-free, egg-free, vegetarian, vegan, and kid-friendly. Low Carb Yum has something for everyone and is an excellent resource if you have any food allergies or sensitivities.

FatForWeightLoss

Aaron Day is an accredited nutritional therapist, advanced sports exercise nutritional adviser, and clinical weight loss practitioner. On his site (www.fatforweightloss.com.au), he leverages his background to create recipes that are low-carb while prioritizing overall health and well-being instead of just weight loss. Aaron believes that you should have ambitious goals that push you past what society deems possible, and food is a critical cornerstone of doing just that.

FatForWeightLoss is filled with recipes and an interactive "Keto FAQ" section where Aaron responds directly to your questions. If you're curious about some aspect of low-carb dieting and need an expert opinion, his site is an excellent resource.

Wellness Mama

WellnessMama (www.wellnessmama.com) is an online community founded by Katie Wells. Although her resources can usually be applied to anyone, she specifically focuses on helping women and moms live a healthier life. Food is undoubtedly a part of that, but it's so much more. You can find everything here, from medical advice (any medical recommendations are reviewed and approved by a group of doctors and medical advisors) to life tips like creating natural deodorant. Complete with a blog and podcast, this site is a tremendous, positive resource for women and moms in particular.

Chocolate Covered Katie

Katie's favorite food is chocolate, and it may be fair to say her life revolves around it! She believes in eating dessert every single day while balancing it so your sweet tooth and overall health are both treated well. Her site (www.chocolatecovered katie.com) is among the top 25 cooking websites on the Internet and the top source for healthy desserts. It's chock-full of sweet and nutritious dishes; she has more categories than some food blogs have recipes. This is a must-have resource for anyone who wants to live healthy and make dessert a central part of that.

Sugar-Free Londoner

Katrin Nürnberger was born in Germany and moved to London in her 20s, so her passion for food has a European twist that's hard to replicate from American-based sites. Her food journey began with a tough medical diagnosis that proved nearly impossible to treat. After months of appointments and round after round of antibiotics, she finally found her answer in a sugar detox. Systemic, sugar-fed inflammation had wreaked havoc on her life, and a low-carb lifestyle rejuvenated her.

Her site (www.sugarfreelondoner.com) is filled with recipes and packed with informational articles covering everything from diet app reviews to step-by-step meal-planning instructions. If you want an in-depth discussion about why you should consider going low-carb, this resource needs to be on your list.

Kalyn's Kitchen

Kalyn Denny's journey into food-based fitness began in 2005. She lost 40 pounds and was so excited about her success that she started blogging about it, which quickly developed into a full-time passion. Kalyn's site (www.kalynskitchen.com) is unique because it doesn't focus exclusively, or even primarily, on keto. She describes her recipes as "carb-conscious" and has individual sections for major diets, including paleo, South Beach, gluten-free, dairy-free, meatless, and vegan. The layout is intuitive and easy to use, allowing you to search for recipes by diet type, category, or ingredients.

Kalyn was a teacher for 30 years, and this life experience shines through in everything she writes. She doesn't stop with simple recommendations and follows up with an explanation of why you should be doing it. If you're curious about the intersection of multiple diets, make sure you thoroughly explore Kalyn's Kitchen.

Ditch the Carbs

Ditch the Carbs (www.ditchthecarbs.com) is focused on transitioning newcomers out of a high-carb diet and into the low-carb lifestyle. The "How to Start" section will walk you through low-carb living step by step, beginning with the why behind keto. It also breaks down high-level concepts into tangible actions you can immediately incorporate into your life.

One of the unique aspects of this site is its section on going low-carb for kids. This can be a significant speed bump for many parents, with questions about whether low-carb, high-fat (LCHF) dieting is safe for kids, how to implement it effectively, and how to make it palatable. If your diet journey involves children, this site should be on your bookmarks list.

Joy Filled Eats

Taryn loves to tell people that she lost 50 pounds and enjoyed every bite. As a mother of six, she found that her baby weight never totally disappeared — in fact, it increased after each child. By the time her fourth child had been born, she'd had enough — that decision eventually led to Joy Filled Eats (www.joyfilledeats.com).

Her philosophy closely aligns with ours: eating healthy and losing weight shouldn't be a painful process. Food is enjoyable, and it shouldn't be any less delicious because it's good for you. All her recipes are sugar- and gluten-free, so if these areas are dietary concerns for you, thoroughly exploring her site should be a top priority.

Hey Keto Mama

Sam Dillard believes that keto is only part of the picture and that spiritual and mental health are just as important. She doesn't see them as separate, disconnected pieces, but rather three parts of a whole that interact and combine to create a healthy you. As a wife and mother, she's intimately familiar with the daily stress and pressures that come with raising a family. All her recipes and diet advice at www.heyketomama.com keep this perspective at the forefront. If you want an honest look at what low-carb living looks like in a family context, this resource is a must-see.

Appendix

Metric Conversion Guide

Note: The recipes in this book weren't developed or tested using metric measurements. There may be some variation in quality when converting to metric units.

Common Abbreviations

Abbreviation(s)	What It Stands For
cm	Centimeter
C., c.	Cup
G, g	Gram
kg	Kilogram
L, l	Liter
lb.	Pound
mL, ml	Milliliter
oz.	Ounce
pt.	Pint
t., tsp.	Teaspoon
T., Tb., Tbsp.	Tablespoon

Volume

U.S. Units	Canadian Metric	Australian Metric
¼ teaspoon	1 milliliter	1 milliliter
½ teaspoon	2 milliliters	2 milliliters
1 teaspoon	5 milliliters	5 milliliters
1 tablespoon	15 milliliters	20 milliliters
¼ cup	50 milliliters	60 milliliters
⅓ cup	75 milliliters	80 milliliters
½ cup	125 milliliters	125 milliliters
⅔ cup	150 milliliters	170 milliliters
¾ cup	175 milliliters	190 milliliters
1 cup	250 milliliters	250 milliliters
1 quart	1 liter	1 liter
1½ quarts	1.5 liters	1.5 liters
2 quarts	2 liters	2 liters
2½ quarts	2.5 liters	2.5 liters
3 quarts	3 liters	3 liters
4 quarts (1 gallon)	4 liters	4 liters

Weight

U.S. Units	Canadian Metric	Australian Metric
1 ounce	30 grams	30 grams
2 ounces	55 grams	60 grams
3 ounces	85 grams	90 grams
4 ounces (¼ pound)	115 grams	125 grams
8 ounces (½ pound)	225 grams	225 grams
16 ounces (1 pound)	455 grams	500 grams (½ kilogram)

Length

Inches	Centimeters
0.5	1.5
1	2.5
2	5.0
3	7.5
4	10.0
5	12.5
6	15.0
7	17.5
8	20.5
9	23.0
10	25.5
11	28.0
12	30.5

Temperature (Degrees)

Fahrenheit	Celsius
32	0
212	100
250	120
275	140
300	150
325	160
350	180
375	190
400	200
425	220
450	230
475	240
500	260

Index

About the Authors

Rami and Vicky Abrams are two entrepreneurs based in Brooklyn, New York. They were first introduced to the keto diet in 2014 and were initially (and understandably) a bit skeptical about a diet that allowed them to eat more butter and bacon than whole grains. However, their curiosity slowly got the better of them, and they dug deep into the diet's background. They were impressed by what they found: at every turn, medical experts and peer-reviewed studies backed up keto's claims. They decided to give it a try, and within just a few weeks, they were dropping pounds and had never felt healthier.

Every other diet they'd tried or seen friends struggle through seemed to be characterized by difficulty. It was almost as if losing weight was meant to be a painful experience, but with keto, that trend reversed itself. The number on the scale seemed to go down effortlessly, but that wasn't even the best part. As they went farther in their keto journey, they realized that their energy was steady throughout the day. They didn't experience the ups and downs between meals or the "hangriness" when they'd gone too long without eating. In fact, it wasn't uncommon for them to unintentionally skip meals because they just forgot to eat. They also realized that brain fog was almost a thing of the past; their mental clarity and ability to be present throughout the day reached levels they'd never felt before. What started as a short-term experiment driven by curiosity turned into a complete life transformation.

Both Rami and Vicky are self-professed foodies who love to try new dishes and types of food at every opportunity. Although enamored with their newfound way of fat-focused cooking and all the flavors it provided, they found that they were missing many of their old favorites. Determined to have their (low-carb) cake and eat it, too, they began to seek out new ways of re-creating established conventions in the kitchen.

Doing so involved a bit of trial and error (and a few rather loud encounters with the smoke detector), but eventually, they cracked the code and never looked back. Vicky loves to say that there are ways of re-creating nearly all your favorite foods, including dessert. For a diet that revolves around eliminating processed sugar and other harmful sweeteners, that's quite the achievement.

At the start of 2015, Rami and Vicky developed Tasteaholics.com. They focused on two things: writing articles filled with medical, scientific, and dietary data while also creating and photographing recipes and then blogging about their progress. The site rapidly became known as both a trendsetter within the keto community and an expert source for both keto information and tantalizing recipes. By the second year, they began publishing their popular series of cookbooks called *Keto in Five*. The cookbooks revolve around three basic principles: every recipe contains five or fewer grams of net carbs per serving, consists of five or fewer ingredients, and can be prepared in five easy steps. Between their website and cookbooks, they were so successful that they were able to quit their jobs and focus exclusively on Tasteaholics.

In 2017, the Abrams launched So Nourished, Inc., a company dedicated to creating keto-friendly ingredients and products, such as healthy sugar replacements and low-carb brownies, pancake mixes, and syrups. At the same time, they expanded their sites to include meal plans and keto-focused news articles, and then launched the Total Keto Diet mobile app. In 2019, the Abrams released *Keto Diet For Dummies*, which quickly became a top-selling keto diet book and resource.

Although they stay busy, the Abrams made plenty of time to engage in two of their favorite activities: trying new food and traveling. They spent six months exploring eight different countries, sampling each area's delicacies, and blogging about the keto lifestyle and low-carb recipes from around the globe. As the healthy fat revolution continues, Rami and Vicky remain dedicated to sharing their experiences with the benefits of ketosis in every area of their lives.

Dedication

To our global keto family, you are the reason we do what we do. You inspire us. The positive energy we see every day on social media fuels our innovation, and the encouragement we regularly find in our inboxes shows that you've become the family we never knew we needed. We're grateful you were willing to ask questions, explore new territory, and relentlessly demand both health *and* flavor!

Authors' Acknowledgments

In writing this book, we are indebted to numerous experts, researchers, and fellow low-carb pioneers who have tirelessly worked to discover the truth.

Our dear friend Yuriy Petriv was our earliest keto diet influencer, introducing us not only to the ketogenic lifestyle but also to each other! His friendship and partnership (in So Nourished, Inc.) have been cornerstones of our personal and business efforts from the very beginning.

Josh Burnett, our chief editor at Tasteaholics and So Nourished, acted as an invaluable guide who shaped large portions of this book with his timely feedback and proactive and detailed guidance.

Writing this book wouldn't have been possible without Tracy Boggier, senior acquisitions editor at Wiley, who brought this project to us. We want to thank the entire team of editors who worked on this book: Chad Sievers (project editor) and Emily Nolan (recipe tester and nutrition analyst).

Publisher's Acknowledgments

Senior Acquisition Editor: Tracy Boggier

Project and Copy Editor: Chad R. Sievers

Recipe Tester and Nutritional Analyst:
Emily Nolan

Production Editor: Tamilmani Varadharaj

Cover Image and Photography:
© Irina Sumchenko/Wiley

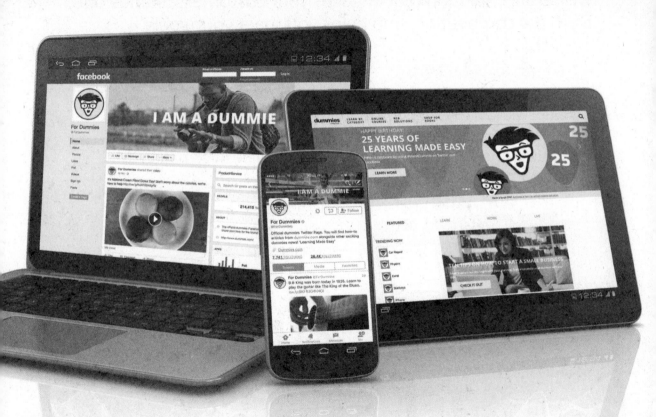

Take dummies with you everywhere you go!

Whether you are excited about e-books, want more from the web, must have your mobile apps, or are swept up in social media, dummies makes everything easier.

Find us online!

     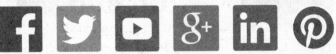

Leverage the power

Dummies is the global leader in the reference category and one of the most trusted and highly regarded brands in the world. No longer just focused on books, customers now have access to the dummies content they need in the format they want. Together we'll craft a solution that engages your customers, stands out from the competition, and helps you meet your goals.

Advertising & Sponsorships

Connect with an engaged audience on a powerful multimedia site, and position your message alongside expert how-to content. Dummies.com is a one-stop shop for free, online information and know-how curated by a team of experts.

- Targeted ads
- Video
- Email Marketing
- Microsites
- Sweepstakes sponsorship

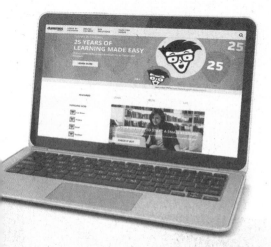

20 MILLION PAGE VIEWS EVERY SINGLE MONTH

15 MILLION UNIQUE VISITORS PER MONTH

43% OF ALL VISITORS ACCESS THE SITE VIA THEIR MOBILE DEVICES

700,000 NEWSLETTER SUBSCRIPTIONS TO THE INBOXES OF

300,000 UNIQUE INDIVIDUALS EVERY WEEK

# of dummies

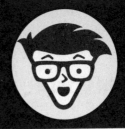

Custom Publishing

Reach a global audience in any language by creating a solution that will differentiate you from competitors, amplify your message, and encourage customers to make a buying decision.

- Apps
- Books
- eBooks
- Video
- Audio
- Webinars

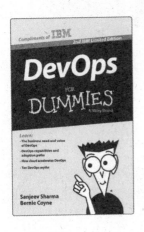
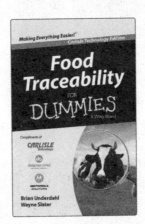
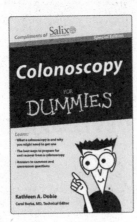
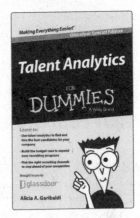

Brand Licensing & Content

Leverage the strength of the world's most popular reference brand to reach new audiences and channels of distribution.

For more information, visit **dummies.com/biz**

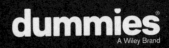

PERSONAL ENRICHMENT

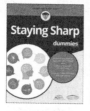

Staying Sharp
9781119187790
USA $26.00
CAN $31.99
UK £19.99

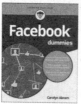

Facebook
9781119179030
USA $21.99
CAN $25.99
UK £16.99

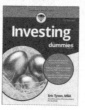

Guitar
9781119293354
USA $24.99
CAN $29.99
UK £17.99

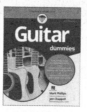

Investing
9781119293347
USA $22.99
CAN $27.99
UK £16.99

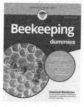

Beekeeping
9781119310068
USA $22.99
CAN $27.99
UK £16.99

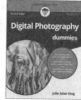

Digital Photography
9781119235606
USA $24.99
CAN $29.99
UK £17.99

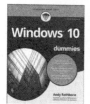

Meditation
9781119251163
USA $24.99
CAN $29.99
UK £17.99

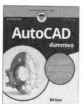

Pregnancy
9781119235491
USA $26.99
CAN $31.99
UK £19.99

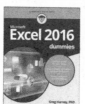

Samsung Galaxy S7
9781119279952
USA $24.99
CAN $29.99
UK £17.99

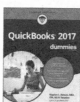

iPhone
9781119283133
USA $24.99
CAN $29.99
UK £17.99

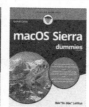

Crocheting
9781119287117
USA $24.99
CAN $29.99
UK £16.99

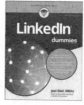

Nutrition
9781119130246
USA $22.99
CAN $27.99
UK £16.99

PROFESSIONAL DEVELOPMENT

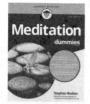

Windows 10
9781119311041
USA $24.99
CAN $29.99
UK £17.99

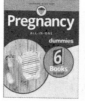

AutoCAD
9781119255796
USA $39.99
CAN $47.99
UK £27.99

Excel 2016
9781119293439
USA $26.99
CAN $31.99
UK £19.99

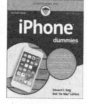

QuickBooks 2017
9781119281467
USA $26.99
CAN $31.99
UK £19.99

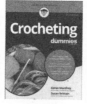

macOS Sierra
9781119280651
USA $29.99
CAN $35.99
UK £21.99

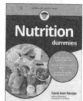

LinkedIn
9781119251132
USA $24.99
CAN $29.99
UK £17.99

Windows 10
9781119310563
USA $34.00
CAN $41.99
UK £24.99

SharePoint 2016
9781119181705
USA $29.99
CAN $35.99
UK £21.99

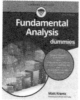

Fundamental Analysis
9781119263593
USA $26.99
CAN $31.99
UK £19.99

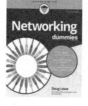

Networking
9781119257769
USA $29.99
CAN $35.99
UK £21.99

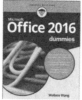

Office 2016
9781119293477
USA $26.99
CAN $31.99
UK £19.99

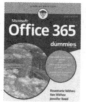

Office 365
9781119265313
USA $24.99
CAN $29.99
UK £17.99

Salesforce.com
9781119239314
USA $29.99
CAN $35.99
UK £21.99

Coding
9781119293323
USA $29.99
CAN $35.99
UK £21.99

dummies.com

dummies
A Wiley Brand

Learning Made Easy

ACADEMIC

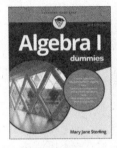

Algebra I dummies

Mary Jane Sterling

9781119293576
USA $19.99
CAN $23.99
UK £15.99

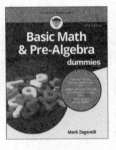

Basic Math & Pre-Algebra dummies

Mark Zegarelli

9781119293637
USA $19.99
CAN $23.99
UK £15.99

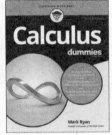

Calculus dummies

Mark Ryan

9781119293491
USA $19.99
CAN $23.99
UK £15.99

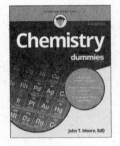

Chemistry dummies

John T. Moore, EdD

9781119293460
USA $19.99
CAN $23.99
UK £15.99

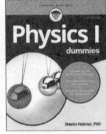

Physics I dummies

Steven Holzner, PhD

9781119293590
USA $19.99
CAN $23.99
UK £15.99

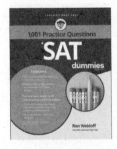

1,001 Practice Questions
SAT dummies

Ron Woldoff

9781119215844
USA $26.99
CAN $31.99
UK £19.99

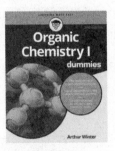

Organic Chemistry I dummies

Arthur Winter

9781119293378
USA $22.99
CAN $27.99
UK £16.99

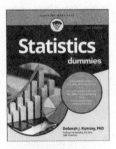

Statistics dummies

Deborah J. Rumsey, PhD

9781119293521
USA $19.99
CAN $23.99
UK £15.99

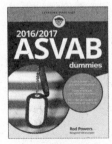

2016/2017
ASVAB dummies

Rod Powers

9781119239178
USA $18.99
CAN $22.99
UK £14.99

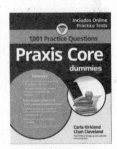

Includes Online Practice Tests
1,001 Practice Questions
Praxis Core dummies

Carla Kirkland
Chan Cleveland

9781119263883
USA $26.99
CAN $31.99
UK £19.99

Available Everywhere Books Are Sold

dummies.com

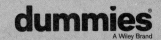

Small books for big imaginations

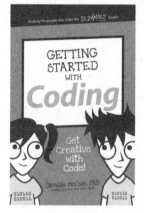
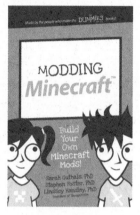
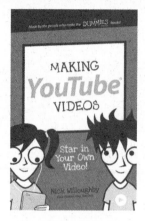
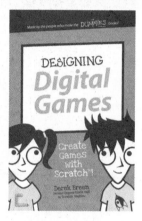
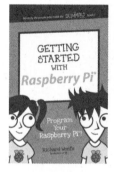
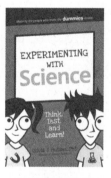
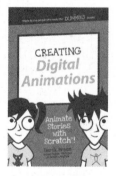
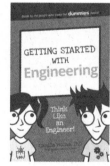
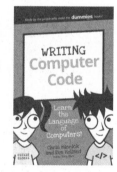
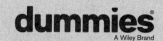